HEART TRANSPLANTATION IN CHILDREN

Edited by

Jeffrey M. Dunn, M.D.
Professor of Surgery
Temple University
School of Medicine;
Director, Pediatric Heart Institute
St. Christopher's Hospital for Children,
Philadelphia, Pennsylvania

Richard M. Donner, M.D.
Associate Professor of Pediatrics
Temple University School of Medicine;
Director, Pediatric Heart Institute
St. Christopher's Hospital for Children,
Philadelphia, Pennsylvania

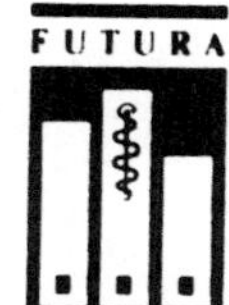

Futura Publishing Company, Inc.
Mount Kisco, NY
1990

Library of Congress Cataloging-in-Publication Data

Heart transplantation in children / edited by Jeffrey M. Dunn.
p. cm.
Includes bibliographical references.
ISBN 0-87993-364-X
1. Heart—Transplantation. 2. Children—Surgery. I. Dunn, Jeffrey M.
[DNLM: 1. Heart—transplantation. 2. Heart Diseases—in infancy & childhood. WS 290 H4362]
RD598.35.T7H43 1990
617.4′120592—dc20
DNLM/DLC
for Library of Congress 89-23834
CIP

Published by
Futura Publishing Company, Inc
P.O. Box 330
Mount Kisco, New York 10549

L.C. No.: 89-23834
ISBN No.: 0-87993-364-X

Printed in the United States of America

Dedicated to
David, Kathryn,
Rachel, and Joshua

Contributors

Terry M. Anderson, M.D. Assistant Professor of Pediatrics, Temple University School of Medicine, Director, Echocardiography Laboratory, St. Christopher's Hospital for Children, Philadelphia, Pennsylvania

Rohinton K. Balsara, M.D. Professor of Surgery, Temple University School of Medicine, Philadelphia, Pennsylvania

Henry T. Bahnson, M.D. Professor of Surgery, University of Pittsburgh School of Medicine, Pittsburgh, Pennsylvania

David Baum, M.D. Professor of Pediatrics, Chief, Division of Pediatric Cardiology, Stanford University School of Medicine, Stanford, California

Lee B. Beerman, M.D. Associate Professor of Pediatrics, University of Pittsburgh, Pittsburgh, Pennsylvania

Daniel Bernstein, M.D. Assistant Professor of Pediatrics, Division of Pediatric Cardiology, Stanford University School of Medicine, Stanford, California

David A. Burton, M.D. Assistant Professor Of Pediatrics, Temple University School of Medicine, Philadelphia, Pennsylvania

Nicholas C. Cavarocchi, M.D. Associate Professor of Surgery, Wayne State University School of Medicine, Director, Cardiopulmonary Transplantation, Harper Hospital, Detroit, Michigan

Craig R. Cohen, M.D. Assistant Professor of Surgery, Temple University School of Medicine, Philadelphia, Pennsylvania

Catherine A. Cooney, B.S.N. Delaware Valley Transplant Program, Philadelphia, Pennsylvania

G. Michael Deeb, M.D. Assistant Professor of Surgery, Director, Cardiac Transplantation and Device Program, University of Michigan Hospital, Ann Arbor, Michigan

Angelo DiGeorge, M.D. Professor of Pediatrics, Temple University School of Medicine, Philadelphia, Pennsylvania

Richard M. Donner, M.D. Associate Professor of Pediatrics, Temple University School of Medicine; Director, Pediatric Heart Institute, St. Christopher's Hospital for Children, Philadelphia, Pennsylvania

Jeffrey M. Dunn, M.D. Professor of Surgery, Temple University School of Medicine; Director, Pediatric Heart Institute, St. Christopher's Hospital for Children, Philadelphia, Pennsylvania

Leona Fields, B.S. University of Pennsylvania, Philadelphia, Pennsylvania

Margaret C. Fisher, M.D. Associate Professor of Pediatrics, Temple University School of Medicine, Philadelphia, Pennsylvania

F. Jay Fricker, M.D. Associate Professor of Pediatrics, University of Pittsburgh School of Medicine, Pittsburgh, Pennsylvania

Bruce I. Goldman, M.D. Associate Professor of Pathology, Temple University School of Medicine, Philadelphia, Pennsylvania

Bartley Griffith, M.D. Professor of Surgery, University of Pittsburgh School of Medicine, Pittsburgh, Pennsylvania

Robert L. Hardesty, M.D. Professor of Surgery, University of Pittsburgh School of Medicine, Pittsburgh, Pennsylvania

Kathy Lawrence, R.N. Clinical Nurse Specialist, University of Pittsburgh School of Medicine, Pittsburgh, Pennsylvania

David A. Lowe, M.D. Associate Professor of Anesthesiology and Pediatrics, Temple University School of Medicine, Philadelphia, Pennsylvania

Constantine Mavroudis, M.D. Professor of Surgery, Northwestern University Medical School, Division Head, Cardiovascular and Transplant Surgery, Children's Memorial Hospital, Chicago, Illinois

James B. McClurken, M.D. Assistant Professor of Surgery, Temple University School of Medicine, Philadelphia, Pennsylvania

Howard M. Nathan, B.S. Executive Director, Delaware Valley Transplant Program, Philadelphia, Pennsylvania

Elfriede Pahl M.D. Associate Professor of Pediatrics, University of Pittsburgh School of Medicine, Pittsburgh, Pennsylvania

Pierantonio Russo, M.D. Assistant Professor of Surgery, Temple University School of Medicine; Director, Pediatric Heart Institute, St. Christopher's Hospital for Children, Philadelphia, Pennsylvania

Leslie M. Shaw, Ph.D. Professor, Department of Pathology and Laboratory Medicine, School of Medicine, University of Pennsylvania; Director, Clinical Toxicology Laboratory, Hospital of the University of Pennsylvania, Philadelphia, Pennsylvania

Vaughn Starnes, M.D. Assistant Professor Of Cardiovascular Surgery, Stanford School of Medicine, Stanford, California

Virginia A. Travitzky, R.N. Delaware Valley Transplant Program, Philadelphia, Pennsylvania

Alfredo Trento, M.D. Assistant Professor of Surgery, University of Pittsburgh School of Medicine, Pittsburgh, Pennsylvania

Carolyn Viewig, R.N., M.S.N. Cardiac Clinical Nurse Specialist, Cooper Medicine, Camden, New Jersey

J.R. Zuberhuhler, M.D. Professor of Pediatric Medicine, University of Pittsburgh School of Medicine, Pittsburgh, Pennsylvania

Preface

With improved survival, cardiac transplantation must now be considered a relatively safe and efficacious tool in the armamentarium of end-stage cardiac disease. Prior to 1980, few cardiac transplants were performed; however, there was a exponential growth during the early 1980s and a consistent, but slower growth in the last few years.* This growth reflects increased confidence in transplantation as an appropriate treatment option and increased organ availability. The slowing of the growth probably reflects the realities of a restrictive donor availability. The Sixth Official Report (1989) of the Registry of the International Society for Heart Transplantation* identifies just under 2450 heart transplants for 1988.

The improved results with cardiac transplantation and growing experience has led to a relaxation of earlier restrictions on cardiac transplantation. Heart transplantation now is routinely offered to young and old candidates. Between 1984 and 1988, 576 transplants in patients under 18 years of age have been reported to the registry. Sixty seven patients were under one year, 125 under five years, and 196 under 10 years of age.

The experience with pediatric transplantation has been gratifying. Although the operative mortality remains higher (25%) in patients under nine years of age compared to the adult population, five-year actuarial survival is not influenced by age. We expect continued expansion of the indications for pediatric cardiac transplantation to include congenital cardiac lesions presently poorly palliated by more conventional procedures.

*Kay M: Sixth Official Report (1989) of the Registry of the International Society for Heart Transplantation. J Heart Transplant, vol. 8, 1989.

Introduction

Heart transplantation is increasingly accepted as effective therapy for end-stage heart disease in children. With increasing experience and improving results, transplantation must be considered in situations where alternate medical and surgical treatment is available but with less than acceptable results. Thus, implementation of cardiac transplantation as therapy for severe structural heart disease currently is debated but strongly favored by some. Technical, medical, and financial difficulties of transplantation have been solved to varying degrees and will continue to diminish. Despite this optimistic outlook, however, pediatric heart transplantation is performed in relatively few centers; experience in any one center is limited by the availability of donor organs. Therefore, the opportunity for firsthand experience with this group of patients may be limited.

This volume is intended to serve two purposes. First, it should serve as an introductory text to all health care professionals who wish to become more familiar with basic concepts. Second, it offers practical suggestions for implementation of a transplant program based upon the experiences, successes, and failures at our institution. The content ranges from a detailed discussion of anesthetic management of the donor and recipient (Chapter 5) to the presentation of sample flow sheets and database forms (Appendix). Although some chapters are more heavily weighted with didactic material and others with practical information, we feel that a satisfactory balance has been achieved. The overall organization begins with pretransplantation considerations, progresses through the peritransplant period, and continues on to discuss chronic management and long-term results. The majority of this text presents the unified approach in use at St. Christopher's Hospital for Children and Temple University in Philadelphia. However, three important chapters (Chapters 7, 15, and 16) have been included to reflect the experiences and thoughts of other programs.

We sincerely hope that this volume will stimulate, encourage, and prepare individuals and institutions interested in establishing a pediatric heart transplant program.

Jeffrey M. Dunn
Richard M. Donner
Philadelphia, Pennsylvania

Contents

Chapter 1

Heart Transplantation Historical Highlights

Rohinton K. Balsara

"Thus said the Lord God...a new heart also will I give you and a new spirit will I put within you; and I will take away the stony heart out of your flesh, and I will give you an heart of flesh." Ezekiel 36:26

The early history of organ transplantation has been related to the human yearning for longevity. In the second century BC, the Chinese surgeons Hua T'o and Pien Chiso had been credited with "swapping" a number of internal organs from their victims while they were sleeping. Another legend has it that the twin brothers Cosmas and Damian,[1] in third century AD, removed a cancerous leg of a white man and replaced it with the leg of a recently deceased Moor.

The earliest record of autogenous pedicled grafts from the forehead, neck, and cheek to restore mutilation of the nose, ear, and lip is found in the Sushruta Shamita, Sanskrit texts of India. Aristotle offered that the heart is the seat of the soul, the emotions, and the intellect, and of immense importance. With their inhibitions, the 14th century physician Gasparo Tagliacozzi[2] argued against transplantation of donor grafts for he felt that such an approach would not only be a physical impossibility but also impractical because of the "force and power" of the individual. It was to be 400 years before that "force and power" was identified as rejection.

The modern revival of interest in transplantation began with John Hunter[3] (1728–1793), who performed xenograft transplants in lower

From *Heart Transplantation in Children*, edited by Jeffrey M. Dunn, M.D. and Richard M. Donner, M.D. © 1990, Futura Publishing Company, Inc., Mount Kisco, NY.

animals. Lister's contribution to antisepsis and subsequent development of asepsis allowed surgical grafting and transplantation to be performed with decreased rate of infection. In the first decade of the 1900s, Charles Guthrie[4] and Alexis Carrel advanced transplantation with their observation: "Unless you can stitch blood vessels together effectively, you can't transplant organs, for organs need an efficient blood supply for its very survival."

The first human organ transplant was accomplished by Voronoy,[5] a Russian, who in 1933 transplanted a kidney on a patient dying of renal failure. The patient survived 48 hours. He attempted six more kidney transplants without success.

The stimulus to continue and consequently the present-day surge of interest in transplant came after World War II with the advent of the "artificial kidney" by Willem Kolff[6] of Holland. Hemodialysis afforded the surgeon a stable retransplant candidate, as well as a backup, should the kidney fail.

A milestone in the understanding of rejection and immunology was reached by Peter Medawar,[7] who in 1944 observed skin graft rejection in burn patients. He and others attempted to suppress skin graft rejection with whole-body radiation and immunosuppressive drugs. For this work, Peter Medawar was awarded the Nobel prize in medicine in 1960. The immunosuppressive drug, antilymphocytic serum (ALS) was first produced by Russian scientist Elie Metchnikoff[8] in 1899, but only in 1963 was it found experimentally to prolong graft longevity.

After early works of Guthrie and Carrel, cardiac transplantation was largely ignored until 1933, when Frank Mann and associates[9] of Rochester, Minnesota stimulated a renewed interest. They embarked on experimentation on heart models to study denervation and cardiac drug activity. Using a canine model with heterotopic transplantation to the neck, they achieved survival of 4–8 days. During the same period, a Russian, Vladimir Demikhov[10] transplanted 250 heterotopic hearts in dogs. In 1958, Gumersindo Blanco and associates[11] reported transplanted hearts in dogs utilizing cardiopulmonary bypass and "cardioplegia" protection.

Surgical modifications made cardiac transplantation more practical. At Guy's Hospital, London, Russel Brock and Henry Cass[12] avoided individual suturing of vena cava and the pulmonary veins by utilizing left and right atrial cuffs. In the United States at the same time, Lower and Shumway[13] were perfecting the technical details introducing the concept of hypothermic protection of the donor heart and far distance procurement of the donor organs. The major obstacle became rejection. Keith Ramstsma[14] of Tulane University increased the survival time of 10 days (control animals) to 27 days in animals treated with methotrexate. Azathioprine and total body-dose radiation of the donor organs also improved graft survival.

Adrian Kantrowitz and his colleagues[15] in 1964 achieved prolonged graft survival by transplanting immature hearts into adult dogs without the use of any immunosuppression, demonstrating less rejection and heart growth.

In 1964, the first human heart transplant was performed by James Hardy and associates[16] at the University of Mississippi, utilizing a chimpanzee donor heart. The chimpanzee heart failed because of severe donor–recipient size mismatch.

On December 2, 1967 Christian Barnard[17] performed the first human allograft heart transplant using the heart of a brain-dead donor. The recipient was Louis Washkansky, a 54-year-old diabetic with a history of two previous heart attacks and an irreparably damaged heart. The donor was a 24-year-old girl with head injury. Immunosuppression was managed with steroids, azathioprine, and local cardiac irradiation. Washkansky died 13 days postoperatively with pulmonary infection. At necropsy, cardiac rejection was absent. Within days of Barnard's success, Adrian Kantrowitz in New York performed a heart transplant on a baby 2½ weeks old with a lethal congenital heart defect. The donor in this case was an anencephalic neonate. The recipient survived for 6 hours.

Barnard attempted a second heart transplantation on January 2, 1968. The recipient Phillip Blaiberg, survived 593 days, successfully overcoming multiple rejection crises. Cardiac transplant interest increased tremendously as did the medicolegal issue of brain death. Ethics committees in medical societies and legislatures redefined "death" and established criteria for organ donation. In the 20 months after the first human heart transplantation, 143 transplantations were performed worldwide. Only 29 of these 143 survived beyond 6 months. Disappointed by poor results, lack of donors, and tremendous costs, only 10 of the 56 teams involved in the initial flurry of activity continued to perform transplants.[18]

With the introduction of cyclosporin, multiple centers again began heart transplantation. The expected 1-year survival rate for heart recipients is now about 85%. It is estimated that in the U.S. alone, 15,000 to 25,000 patients can be considered potential transplant recipients.

In December 1982, an artificial heart was inserted in Dr. Barney Clarke, a 62-year-old dentist suffering from terminal and irreversible heart failure, In Salt Lake City, Utah, a team headed by William DeVries[19] implanted a Jarvik-7 mechanical heart driven by pneumatic pump. The patient survived over 3 months. With the many complications and failures associated with the use of permanent artificial hearts, attention was turned to their use as a "bridge" to transplantation[20,21] in patients who could not be maintained medically prior to transplantation.

In 1987, Baumgartner and his associates[22] performed the first "domino" transplant, in which a patient suffering from cystic fibrosis received a heart–lung transplant and his healthy heart was removed and implanted simultaneously into another patient requiring a new heart.

The first xenograft heart transplant was in 1964 by Hardy and associates, utilizing a chimpanzee heart.[16] Since then, sporadic cases have been reported by Barnard and others, but enthusiasm for xenografts waned as allografts became a routine. In 1984, Leonard Bailey and associates[23] performed a neonatal xenotransplant utilizing a baboon heart for "Baby Fae," who was suffering from hypoplastic left heart syndrome. This represented the first attempt at clinical xenotransplant using cyclosporine as an immunosuppressive agent. Although this transplant was performed across ABO blood barrier, the recipient survived for 21 days before the donor heart was rejected. Extensive experimental work by Bailey has shown that xenograft transplants from lambs to goats could survive for up to 72 days when treated with cyclosporine. Xenografting may be feasible because of the great similarities in the serum proteins, hemoglobin structure, and major blood groups between primates and man. This hopefully could permit in the future successful transplantation across barriers of histocompatibility previously forbidden to man.

The future of cardiac transplantation in children is confirmed by the solid history of transplantation over the past 25 years. With increased improvement of surgical techniques and immunosuppression, the role of cardiac transplantation in children will continue to grow.

References

1. Lyons AS, Petrucelli RJ: Medicine—An Illustrated History. Harry N. Abrams Inc., New York, 1978.
2. Flye MW: History of transplantation. In Flye MW: Principles of Organ Transplantation. W.B. Saunders Co., Philadelphia, 1989, p. 5.

3. Flye MW: History of transplantation. In Flye MW: Principles of Organ Transplantation. W.B. Saunders Co., Philadelphia, 1989, p. 6.
4. Richardson RG: The Scalpel and the Surgeon. Charles Scribner's Sons, New York, 1970, Chapt. 29.
5. Tilney NL, Kirkman RL: Surgical aspects of kidney transplant. In Garovoy MR, Guttmann RD: Renal Transplantation. Churchill Livingstone, New York, 1986, p.93.
6. Kolff WJ, Berk HTR: The artificial kidney: A dialyser with a great area. Acta Med Scand 1944, 117:121.
7. Medawar PB: The behavior & fate of skin autografts & skin homografts in rabbits. J Anat 1944, 78:176.
8. Flye MW: Principles of Organ Transplantation. W.B. Saunders Co., Philadelphia, 1989, Chapt. 1.
9. Mann FC, Priestley JT, Markowitz J, et al: Transplantation of the intact mammalian heart. Arch Surg 1933, 26:219.
10. Demikhov VP: trans. by Haigh B: Experimental Transplantation of Vital Organs. Consultants Bureau, New York, 1962.
11. Blanco G, Adam A, Rodriguez-Perez D: Complete homotransplantation of canine heart & lungs. Arch Surg 1958, 76:20.
12. Cass MH, Brock R: Heart excision and replacement. Guy's Hosp Rep 1959, 108:235.
13. Lower RR, Shumway NE: Studies on orthotopic homo-transplantation of canine heart. Surg Forum 1960, 11:18.
14. Richardson RG: The Scalpel and the Heart. Charles Scribner's Sons, New York, 1970, Chapt. 29.
15. Kondo Y, Gradel F, Kantrowitz A: Homotransplantation of the heart in puppies under profound hypothermia: Long survival without immunosuppressive treatment. Ann Surg 1965, 162:837.
16. Hardy JD, Chavez CM, Kurrus FD, et al: Heart transplantation in man. JAMA 1965, 114:1132.
17. Barnard CN: A human cardiac transplant: An interim report of a successful operation performed at Groote Schuur Hospital, Capetown S. Africa. Med J, 1967, 41:1271.
18. Cooley DA, Bloodwell RD, Hallman GL, et al: Cardiac transplantation: General considerations & results. Ann Thorac Surg 1969, 169:893.
19. Cowart VS: Improvements predicted in artificial heart by 1990—Medical news. JAMA 1985, 253:2621.
20. Copeland JG, Levinson MM, Smith R, et al: The total artificial heart as a bridge to transplantation—Report of two cases. JAMA 1986, 256:2991.
21. Pierce W: Artificial hearts and blood pumps in the treatment of profound heart failure. Circulation 1983, 68:882.
22. Copeland JG, Emery RW: History of cardiothoracic transplantation. Cardiac Surgery: State of Art Review 1988, 2:535.
23. Bailey LL, Nehlsen-Cannarella SL, Concepcion W, et al: Baboon-to-human cardiac xenotransplantation in a neonate. JAMA 1985, 254:3321.
24. Bell E, Ehrlich HP, Buttle DJ, et al: Living tissue formed in vitro and accepted as skin—Equivalent tissue of full thickness. Science 1952, 211: 1052.

Chapter 2

Indications and Candidacy for Heart Transplantation in Children

Terry M. Anderson

The selection of a candidate for heart transplantation is a difficult and many times controversial issue. Since the first human heart transplant over 20 years ago,[1] the indications and contraindications for candidacy have been changing continuously. The selection criteria used 5 years ago are considerably different than those used today and will undoubtedly differ again 5 years from now.

The introduction of cyclosporine in the early 1980s revitalized heart transplantation.[2] Along with this revitalization came major changes in the selection of candidates. The improved outcome and long-term survival associated with cyclosporine were responsible for a relaxation of the medical, psychosocial, and ethical criteria used to select candidates for transplantation. Controversies over age, cardiac functional status, and which systemic diseases should be considered contraindications have led to considerable variation in the selection criteria among heart transplant programs. Today, a candidate for heart transplantation is somewhere in the wide spectrum between being too sick to benefit to being too healthy to be considered. Actual transplantations for this increasing number of qualified candidates, however,

From *Heart Transplantation in Children,* edited by Jeffrey M. Dunn, M.D. and Richard M. Donner, M.D. © 1990, Futura Publishing Company, Inc., Mount Kisco, NY.

are limited by donor organ availability[3] and improved medical and surgery therapy.

Guidelines

The proper selection of an infant, child, or adolescent for heart transplantation may be the most important factor in determining outcome and long-term survival. The selection process is complex and requires that indications be fulfilled and that patients with contraindications be excluded.[4–8] The general indication for transplantation is a significant cardiac disability in the presence of end-stage heart disease (Table 1). The guidelines call for a limited life expectancy despite maximal medical and surgical therapy. The length of life expectancy is no longer as important as it once was. The improved outcome and long-term survival have made transplantation a viable alternative even early in the disease process. An understanding of the prognosis, natural history, and response to treatment of the underlying heart disease is a very important aspect in the selection process.

The New York Heart Association classification system provides a basis for determining the severity of a cardiac disability.[9] In most adult transplant centers, a Class IV disability is considered a criterion for candidate selection. Obviously, it is difficult to apply this classification system to infants and young children. Many candidates, in addition, may not have reached this degree of disability when the decision to transplant is made. No longer does one have to be near death to be considered an acceptable candidate. Patients with end-stage heart disease, who are expected to deteriorate with time, will be better candidates earlier rather than later.[10] Clinical judgment and prognostication are key factors in the proper assessment of a patient for candidacy.

Table 1 Guidelines for Candidate Selection

End-stage heart disease
Limited life expectancy
New York Heart Association Class IV disability
Failure of medical therapy
Exclusion of contraindications

Indications

The indications for heart transplantation in pediatric patients involve both acquired and congenital end-stage heart disease (Table 2).[11–13]

Table 2 Indications for Heart Transplantation

Acquired heart disease
Dilated cardiomyopathy
Hypertrophic cardiomyopathy
Ischemic cardiomyopathy
Life-threatening arrhythmias
Nonmalignant cardiac tumors
Congenital heart disease
Defects not amenable to further surgery
Ventricular pump failure
Alternative surgical procedure

Acquired Heart Disease

The most common acquired end-stage heart disease in children and adolescents is a dilated cardiomyopathy.[13] This is an irreversible cardiomyopathy without known cause or effective therapy. Symptomatic treatment for these patients is not effective and heart transplantation may be indicated. If an etiology for the cardiomyopathy, such as a disorder of carnitine metabolism, is known and therapy is possible, then the specific therapy may be effective and transplantation may not be indicated. It is important, therefore, that a complete and comprehensive search for an etiology be made. More often than not, the etiology will be unknown or the cause untreatable. However, not all idiopathic dilated cardiomyopathies will require transplantation. The severity, age of onset, and potential for improvement are all key determinants in the decision process. An infant with a mild dilated cardiomyopathy will have a better chance at recovery than an older child with a severe cardiomyopathy.[14]

An ischemic cardiomyopathy as a result of coronary artery disease is common in the adult experience,[4,6,7] but uncommon in pediatrics. A rare child may present with an infarction and severely impaired function from an anomalous left coronary artery or a thrombosed coronary artery aneurysm in Kawasaki disease. These patients may be potential candidates for heart transplantation if medical or surgical therapy is ineffective.

Hypertrophic obstructive cardiomyopathies may also be severe enough to necessitate transplantation. The patient with severely impaired diastolic compliance and congestive heart failure may exhibit arrhythmias that do not respond to conventional therapy. In the presence of significant hemodynamic compromise, these arrhythmias will be life threatening. Our transplant experience involves one infant with a severe hypertrophic cardiomyopathy, who developed life-threatening atrial arrhythmias. The arrhythmia was unresponsive to conventional medical therapy and heart transplantation was indicated.

Nonmalignant cardiac tumors, such as fibromas and rhabdomyomas, are unusual forms of end-stage heart disease. Candidates for heart transplantation have tumor mass extensive enough to either impair blood flow and function or produce life-threatening arrhythmias. These tumors are not amenable to surgical resection. In our transplant experience, a 5-month-old infant presented with a massive fibroma of the left ventricle with severe compromise of ventricular pump function. Surgical resection of the tumor mass was impossible and transplantation was indicated.

Other less common forms of acquired heart disease, such as a restrictive cardiomyopathy or life-threatening arrhythmias, may be indication for heart transplantation. The guidelines of end-stage heart disease with a limited life expectancy despite maximal medical and surgical therapy must be met.

Congenital Heart Disease

The second major category of end-stage heart disease in the pediatric population is the result of congenital heart defects (Table 2). Transplantation may be indicated in children with structural cardiac defects not amenable to further surgery, in the presence of ventricular pump failure as a result of the defect, or as an alternative approach to a surgical procedure with poor results.

End-stage congenital heart defects that are not amenable to further surgery may be considered indications for heart transplantation.[15,16] Potentially, this could be a catch-all category, but the ma jority of congenital heart defects can be treated successfully by conventional surgery and should not require transplantation.[12] The more complex structural heart defects may be the exception. In either case, no contraindications should be present. Significant abnormalities of the great arteries or venous return may complicate transplantation for technical reasons. Increased pulmonary vascular resistance is a major contraindication to transplantation and, many times, is present as a result of the structural heart defect. The addition of heart–lung transplantation could potentially aid candidates who have developed irreversible pulmonary vascular disease.

Ventricular pump failure as a direct result of the structural defect or, more commonly following surgery, may be considered an indication for heart transplantation. The heart disease is end-stage with a limited life expectancy and attempts at maximal medical therapy are often unsuccessful. As part of our experience, we have performed heart transplantation in three adolescents who developed end-stage ventricular pump failure following mitral valve replacement. All patients failed attempts at aggressive medical therapy and were considered candidates for transplantation.

One of the most controversial indications for transplantation is an alternative approach to a surgical procedure with generally accepted poor results. The most widely discussed example is the newborn with hypoplastic heart syndrome.[12] Many pediatric centers consider heart transplantation an acceptable alternative to attempts at surgical palliation or the certain mortality of not intervening. This approach to the hypoplastic left heart syndrome is exemplified at Loma Linda University Medical Center, where Dr. Leonard Bailey has performed numerous transplantations with excellent results. As the pediatric transplantation experience improves, it is conceivable that it may replace other procedures for congenital heart disease.

As more experience with pediatric transplantation develops and donor organ availability improves, it is certain that indications for transplantation will change. It is conceivable that palliative surgical procedures will be performed for complex congenital heart defects in anticipation of future heart transplantation. Surgical palliation of an infant with hypoplastic left heart syndrome could provide adequate time to secure a donor organ in a less urgent fashion. It is also possible that with improved outcome and long-term survival, heart transplantation may be a better alternative than some conventional congenital heart procedures.

Contraindications

Equally important in the selection of a candidate for heart transplantation is the identification of any contraindications that would alter the outcome or long-term survival.[4,6,7] As the experience and success with heart transplantation continue to improve, the significance of individual contraindications also changes.

Contraindications may be considered either relative or absolute. Relative contraindications are conditions that can be overcome or corrected and will ultimately not affect the outcome of the transplantation. Absolute contraindications, on the other hand, are generally not reversible and will adversely affect the outcome. Patients with absolute contraindications should not be considered as candidates.

Relative Contraindications

There are many relative contraindications to heart transplantation (Table 3). An active infection can be considered a relative contraindication if that infection can be controlled or eliminated. Once treated, plans for transplantation may proceed. Because intercurrent infections in pediatric patients are common, it may be necessary to interrupt a patient's candidacy temporarily until all evidence of infection has disappeared. As a practical matter, close cooperation with the organ procurement system is essential to minimize anxiety that may result from frequent alteration of the candidate list. Aggressive diagnosis and treatment of intercurrent illness, if possible, is essential to optimize donor-recipient matching.

Table 3 Relative Contraindications to Transplantation

Infection
Elevated pulmonary vascular resistance (4–6 units)
Recent pulmonary infarction
Vascular anomalies
Renal dysfunction
Hepatic dysfunction
Psychosocial instability
Alcohol and/or substance abuse
Limited family support
Financial constraints

The accurate measurement of pulmonary vascular resistance is an important factor in determining contraindications. Fixed pulmonary vascular resistance greater than 6 to 8 Wood's units is currently a strong contraindication. Resistance that is elevated and between 4 and 6 units can be considered a relative contraindication, especially if a reduction of the pulmonary artery pressure and resistance can be demonstrated during the administration of 100% inspired oxygen or pulmonary vasodilators. Patients with low pulmonary vascular resistance are considered optimal candidates.

A recent pulmonary embolus or infarction is also considered a relative contraindication because of the likelihood of pulmonary infection or its exacerbation with initiation of immunosuppression. The source of the embolus should be determined and treated appropriately. If pulmonary vascular resistance remains low, transplantation may proceed. Chronic microthrombi to the pulmonary vasculature may also raise pulmonary vascular resistance, but may be silent until the resistance rises above acceptable values.

Another relative contraindication to transplantation is an anomaly of venous return or arterial connection. These vascular anomalies can be technical deterrents to transplantation,[12] particularly in complex congenital heart defects. Modifications of the surgical transplant technique may overcome this problem.

When considering infants for heart transplantation, prematurity and low birth weight may be contraindications. The accepted criteria at Loma Linda University Medical Center is a gestational age greater than 36 weeks and a birth weight greater than 2,200 grams.[17] Values less than these should be considered relative contraindications.

Abnormalities of other organ systems may also be considered relative contraindications if these problems can be corrected and will not adversely affect the outcome of the transplantation. This would include a wide range of potential problems including abnormalities of renal, hepatic and neurologic function. In addition to aggressive medical management of end-stage heart disease, careful assessment and management of other potential problems are essential.

Other relative contraindications to transplantation include psychosocial instability,[18] alcohol and/or substance abuse, limited family support, and financial constraints. These problems may affect transplant outcome adversely and careful assessment is important. Our experience has demonstrated the unfortunate consequences of inadequate family support mechanisms, with the result that this requirement for candidacy is enforced. External support services or alternative care providers are possible answers to these circumstances.

Absolute Contraindications

Absolute contraindications to heart transplantation are irreversible conditions that would adversely affect the outcome and long-term survival (Table 4). A patient with an absolute contraindication should not be considered a candidate for heart transplantation. There are several well-defined conditions and many other indications that potentially could become absolute contraindications. A major blood group incompatibility between the recipient and donor or the presence of a positive cross-match are probably absolute contraindications to transplantation. A fixed pulmonary vascular resistance greater than 6-8 units, determined by careful measurement techniques and repeated a number of times, argues absolutely against candidacy because right ventricular failure will almost surely result despite aggressive medical management in the postoperative period.

The presence of irreversible and progressive renal or hepatic disease is an absolute contraindication because cyclosporine is nephrotoxic and is metabolized in the liver. Other disease processes that would limit the life expectancy or compromise the recovery from transplantation should be considered absolute contraindications. This is a very broad category and is subject to individual interpretation. There is no question that any coexisting metabolic or neoplastic life-threatening disease would be a major deterrent to transplantation. Not as well defined, however, are diseases that are not immediately life threatening. Chronic lung disease and metabolic and genetic diseases associated with a significantly extended life span (e.g., diabetes, late-onset or undefined glycogenosis, muscular dystrophies) are examples.

Table 4 Absolute Contraindications to Transplantation

ABO incompatibility
Positive specific donor-recipient cross-match
Elevated fixed pulmonary vascular resistance (>6–8 units)
Irreversible and progressive renal disease
Irreversible and progressive hepatic disease
Coexisting life threatening diseases
Significant developmental delay (genetic or acquired)

At the present time, it is our procedure to offer transplant to children with these or similar systemic diseases unless the illness will impact directly on graft survival. It has been our custom to exclude children with significant developmental delay from well-defined genetic (e.g., trisomy 21) or acquired causes. Ultimately, these decisions will be governed by the availability of organs and continued ethical debate by both medical and lay groups.

The newborn infant who is being considered for heart transplant presents some unique problems. The long-term consequences of other organ system diseases, such as structural brain abnormalities or poorly defined genetic syndromes, may not be known. Severe metabolic stress, such as persistent acidosis of pH below 7.10 for more than 2 hours or a blood sugar below 20 mg% for more than 30 min, may complicate the clinical status. If a decision for transplant must be made before the sequelae of these abnormalities are fully known, we prefer not to proceed with transplant.

Conclusions

The selection of heart transplant candidates is a complex process. We must accurately identify patients who meet the criteria of a significant heart disability in the presence of end-stage heart disease and decide who should be considered candidates for transplantation.[19] In addition, screening patients for contraindications is a difficult but necessary process. Potential problems arise in the interpretation of coexisting, non-life-threatening disease,[20] and the selection process involves intelligent prognostication and, in some cases, educated guesswork. The optimal use of the limited supply of donor organs and maintenance of reasonable survival rates remains an overriding concern.

References

1. Barnard CN: The Operation. S Afr Med J 1967, 41:1271.
2. Borel JF: Cylcosporine: Historical perspectives. Transplant Proc 1983, 15(Suppl 1):3.
3. Evans RW, Manninen DL, Garrison LP, et al: Donor availability as the primary determinant of future of heart transplantation. JAMA 1986, 255: 1892.

4. Thompson ME: Selection of candidates for cardiac transplantation. Heart Transplant 1983, 3:65.
5. Painvin GA, Frazier OH, Chandler LB, et al: Cardiac transplantation: Indications, procurement, operation and management. Heart Lung 1985, 14:484.
6. Copeland JG, Emery RW, Levinson MM, et al: Selection of patients for cardiac transplantation. Circulation 1987, 75:2.
7. Barnum BE: Selection of patients for heart transplant. Texas Heart Institute 1987, 14:238.
8. Griffith BP, Hardesty RL, Trento A, et al: Five years of heart transplantation in Pittsburgh. J Heart Transplant 1985, 4:489.
9. Criteria Committee, New York Heart Association, Inc.: Diseases of the Heart and Blood Vessels. Nomenclature and Criteria for Diagnosis. 6th Ed., Little, Brown and Co., Boston, 1964.
10. Keogh AM, Baron DW, Hickie JB: Appropriate timing of heart transplantation for patients with cardiomyopathy. Cardiology Board Review 1988, 5:31.
11. Baum D, Stinston EB, Shumway NE: The place for heart transplantation in children. In Godman MJ, ed: Pediatric Cardiology. Churchill Livingston, London, 1981, pp. 741-747.
12. Penkoske PA, Rowe RD, Freedom RM, et al: The future of heart and heart–lung transplantation in children. Heart Transplant 1984, 3:233.
13. Pennington DG, Sarafian J, Swartz M: Heart transplantation in children. Heart Transplant 1985, 4:441.
14. Griffin ML, Hernandez A, Martin TC, et al: Dilated cardiomyopathy in infants and children. J Am Coll Cardiol 1988, 11:139.
15. Reitz BA, Jamieson SW, Gaudiani VA, et al: Method for cardiac transplantation in corrected transposition. J Cardiovasc Surg 1982, 23:293.
16. Pennington DG, Codd JE, Merjavy JP, et al: The expanded use of ventricular bypass systems for severe cardiac failure and as a bridge to cardiac transplantation. Heart Transplant 1983, 3:38.
17. Infant heart transplantation protocol. Loma Linda International Heart Institute. Loma Linda University Medical Center Cardiac Transplant Program. July 1988.
18. Frierson RL, Lippmann SB: Heart transplant candidates rejected on psychiatric indications. Psychosomatic 1987, 28:347.
19. Caplan AL: Equity in the selection of recipients for cardiac transplants. Circulation 1987, 75:10.
20. Merrikin KJ, Overcast TD: Patient selection for heart transplantation: When is a discriminating choice discrimination? J Health Polit Policy Law 1985, 10:7.

Chapter 3

Evaluation of the Pediatric Cardiac Transplantation Candidate

James B. McClurken and G. Michael Deeb

When the patient is referred for evaluation for orthotopic heart transplantation, it is important to determine if the criteria for heart transplantation have been met. Occasionally, further medical management is possible. It is extremely important to evaluate the patient for potential reversibility of either a congenital or acquired cardiac pathologic process. Surgical correction may offer some improvement to certain patients with deteriorating cardiac status who were otherwise thought to be inoperable, and occasionally, some cardiomyopathies are, at least in part, reversible. It is, therefore, of paramount importance for the cardiac transplant team to thoroughly reevaluate the patient's medical status.

It is important to evaluate the patient and the family and support system about the acceptance of heart transplantation as a concept of treatment. Obviously, this entails educating the family and support members about the short-term and long-term aspects of pediatric cardiac transplantation, especially prognosis and side effects of medications.

From *Heart Transplantation in Children,* edited by Jeffrey M. Dunn, M.D. and Richard M. Donner, M.D.

Contraindications

Occasionally, reevaluation of the patient's clinical status will reveal such contraindications as unsuspected renal failure, hepatic failure, pneumonia, or other unsuspected sepsis. The reversibility of organ dysfunction is sometimes unknown and may simply be secondary to low cardiac output.

A factor that must not be overlooked is whether or not the patient has irreversible pulmonary hypertension. A pulmonary vascular resistance of >6 Woods units is generally a contraindication to orthotopic heart transplantation, because the donor right ventricle will fail in this setting. Nitroglycerin and/or amrinone can be utilized to see if the patient's pulmonary hypertension is reactive in a downward fashion. This obviously requires keeping the patient in an intensive care unit with pulmonary artery catheter monitoring to assess reactivity.

Formal Evaluation

A thorough history and physical examination by the cardiology team, cardiothoracic surgical team, and cardiovascular nurse team are performed with specific attention focused on the present level of treatment and the patient's response. For thorough knowledge of the patient's status, it is imperative to have on hand previous hospital records, cardiac catheterization reports, and operative reports.

Chest radiography, including posterior–anterior and lateral views, is needed. Pulmonary function testing is performed when possible. Noninvasive cardiac scanning is frequently utilized along with complete cardiac catheterization of both the right and left heart. Hemodynamic response to pharmacologic manipulation is documented. In cases of unknown etiology, right heart biopsy is frequently performed to document etiology for cardiac decompensation.

Serum biochemical analysis should include the following: complete blood count with differential, electrolyte determination, BUN and creatinine, total bilirubin, alkaline phosphatase, SGOT, SGPT, LDH, 2-hour postprandial blood glucose levels, and creatinine clearance if BUN and creatinine are abnormal; lipid profile and protein levels; urinalysis, and 24-hour urine for protein when the creatinine clearance is significantly abnormal.

Infectious disease evaluation includes particular emphasis on any obvious sign of infection. Skin testing is performed with intermediate PPD, and an anergy panel is placed. If the child is PPD positive, at least INH prophylaxis is administered.

If any infections are present, thorough cultures are obtained, including nasopharyngeal, throat, urine culture and sensitivity, stool for ova and parasites, and cultures of indwelling catheters. A thorough dental examination is performed when appropriate, and dental treatment carried out prior to transplantation.

Routine childhood immunization status is ascertained, and the child is immunized with pneumococcal vaccine and the appropriate influenza vaccine and Hemophilus influenza vaccine.

Titers to varicella virus, Epstein-Barr virus, cytomegalovirus (CMV), hepatitis B, and toxoplasmosis are obtained. If the child is CMV negative, CMV(−) blood is utilized perioperatively, when available. If the child is positive to toxoplasmosis, peritransplant chemical prophylaxis is administered. Human immunodeficiency virus (HIV) status is obtained for the purpose of information and not discrimination. (There has been at least one intentional transplant in a child with HIV infection, whose status was known prior to transplantation for preterminal ischemic cardiomyopathy.)

A serum sample is stored in the immunoserology labs for possible later use in comparing subsequent titers of other potential infectious agents, such as Aspergillus or Candida.

Immunologic assays performed include percent reactive antibodies and, when there are significant reactive antibodies, cytotoxic screen. Type and crossmatch with ABO blood type is performed and, human lymphocyte antigen tissue typing is usually performed for research purposes.

Physical medicine and rehabilitation personnel evaluate the patient for capability for transfer, bed mobility, gait, endurance, range of motion, and motor function, strength, coordination, and balance. It is important to document this preoperatively because the child may become extremely weak awaiting transplantation for a prolonged period while bedridden.

Psychologic and psychiatric evaluations are performed to include Wechsler memory scale testing, Wechsler adult intelligence scale, human figure drawing, Minnesota Multiphasic Personality Inventory for both the patient, when appropriate, and the support/family members. Obviously, these tests cannot be performed on the young child or the neonate.

Social service evaluation of the patient, family, and other support persons is obtained. Proper financial planning and directing the family members to appropriate agencies for assistance is crucial.

Occupational therapy evaluation is obtained to assess the patient for coping strategies, muscle strength, and range of motion, particularly involving the upper extremities. Therapeutic activities can be planned prior to transplantation so they are familiar to the patient after transplantation, thus enhancing cooperation and compliance.

Dietary evaluation assists with obtaining past, present, and ideal diet and weight circumstances. Review of personal resources is again focused upon by either the social worker or a hospital administrative person.

Lastly, patient relations members evaluate the family and support persons for resources to meet basic needs regarding accommodations and meals near the hospital. The health of the family and support persons must be considered. They frequently go through a long, emotionally trying ordeal, and whatever amenities can be offered are usually greatly appreciated by the family.

Conclusions

An interdisciplinary team comprised of representatives of the appropriate, above-mentioned groups, along with a transplant pharmacist, meets to discuss the patient's candidacy. In general, the following three classifications are used:

An *acceptable candidate* is one about whom there is no disagreement that cardiac transplantation is the best form of therapy and no contraindications have been uncovered. The patient is ranked according to the clinical urgency (see UNOS guidelines).

A *qualified acceptable candidate* is a patient considered acceptable if certain criteria are met. This may include clearance of infection, extraction of a tooth, or the final resolution of a particular medical problem. It is important to outline the requirements needed to become an acceptable candidate for both the patient and the referring physicians.

An *unacceptable candidate* is one about whom there is consensus that cardiac transplantation would not be in the patient's best interest. The patient, family, and referring physician obviously need to be fully informed as to how this decision was reached. The family should not be left in a hopeless sense of desperation. Occasionally, the family will seek an additional opinion at another transplant center. When the family requests such an opinion, all the information gathered about the patient should be shared with that center.

See Appendix A for a working summary of this chapter.

Chapter 4

Organ Procurement Process

Virginia A. Travitzky, Catherine A. Cooney, and Howard M. Nathan

Introduction

The limiting factor in pediatric heart transplantation is the availability of donors that match the needs of the waiting recipients. As of June, 1988, there were approximately 35 pediatric patients under the age of 15 awaiting heart or heart/lung transplantation in the United States (Table 1).[1] Donor hearts must come from brain-dead patients of approximately the same size and compatible blood type. The most common causes of death of pediatric and adult organ donors involve trauma-related incidents such as motor vehicle accidents. Infant and neonatal deaths meeting organ donor criteria occur less frequently than in children and adults and under different circumstances (Table 2).[2] Yet, the most crucial need for pediatric donors exists in this younger population. This is evidenced by the high percentage of patients under age 12 months who received heart transplants during 1984–1988. Nearly one-third of the hearts transplanted in children ages newborn to 10 years of age were infants under 12 months of age (Fig. 1).[3] Because the number of pediatric donors within a given region does not often meet the needs of patients waiting in that area, pediatric heart transplantation depends on a nationwide organ procurement and distribution system that secures hearts from donors who may be hundreds of miles from the transplant center.

The successful procurement of a donor heart requires the cooperation of several teams of health care professionals. The growth of transplantation has created a new health care professional—the trans-

From *Heart Transplantation in Children*, edited by Jeffrey M. Dunn, M.D. and Richard M. Donner, M.D. © 1990, Futura Publishing Company, Inc., Mount Kisco, NY.

Table 1 U.S. Pediatric Heart and Heart/Lung Active Waiting List, June 1988

	Candidate Age Groups		
Organ type	0–5	6–10	11–15
Heart	13	5	13
Heart/lung	1	3	2

Source: United Network for Organ Sharing

Table 2 Frequent Causes of Death of Infant Organ Donors

Asphyxia at birth
Sudden Infant Death Syndrome (SIDS)
Intracranial hemorrhage
Child abuse (Shaken Baby Syndrome)
Tumor/CNS abnormalities
Anoxic injuries (drowning, smoke inhalation)

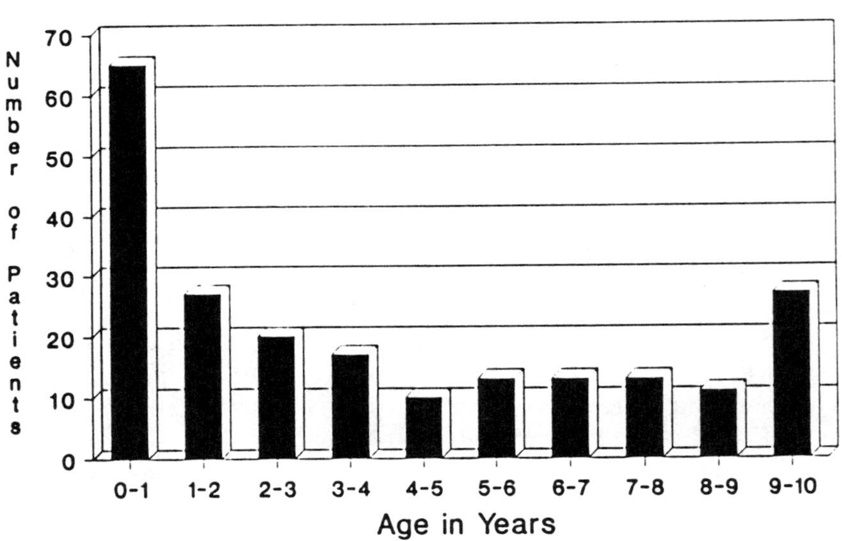

Figure 1: *Heart transplant recipients, age distribution 1984–1988. Source: International Society of Heart Transplantation.*

plant coordinator. The transplant coordinator is responsible for orchestrating the procurement, distribution, preservation, and transportation of organs and tissues.[4]

There are 72 regional organ procurement organizations (OPO) in the U.S., which serve as a conduit between hospitals that provide donor organs and hospitals performing organ transplants. Each OPO has been certified by the Health Care Financing Administration to facilitate organ recovery and donation within a designated area of the U.S. (Fig. 2). Today, all OPO and transplant centers in the United States are members of the National Organ Procurement and Transplantation Network (OPTN) (Fig. 3). The OPTN was established as a result of federal legislation passed in 1984, entitled the National Transplantation Act (PL-508). The contract for the OPTN was awarded to the United Network for Organ Sharing (UNOS) in 1987. UNOS over-

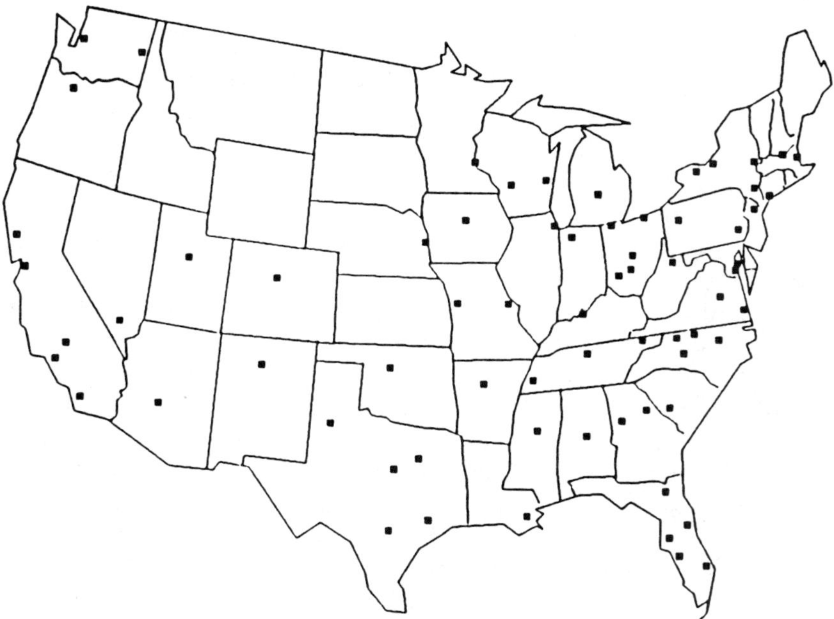

Figure 2: *Location of the 72 U.S. Organ Procurement Organizations (OPO). Sources: Division of Organ Transplantation (DOT); Health Care Financing Administration (HCFA); United Network for Organ Sharing (UNOS).* ■ = *OPO main offices.*

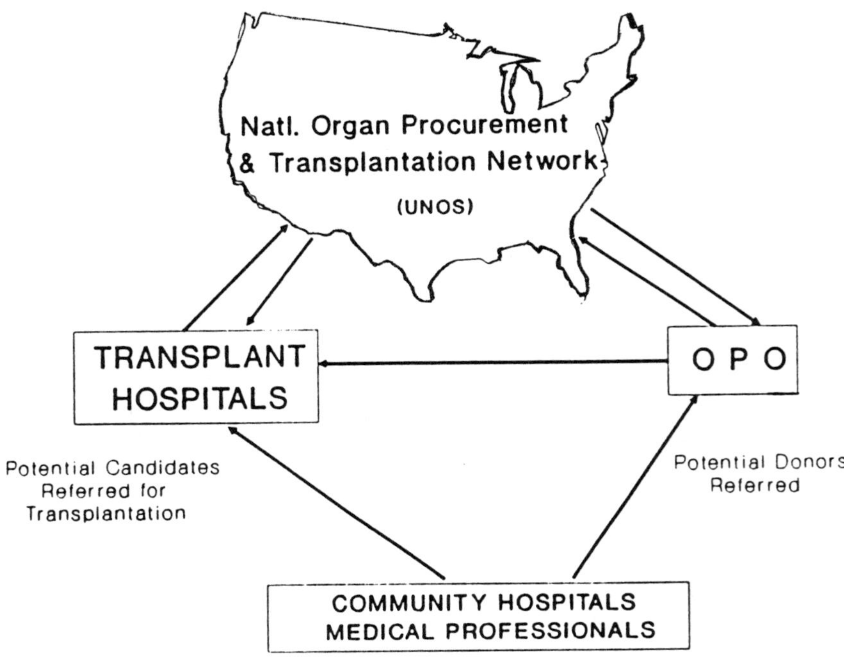

Figure 3: *The U.S. transport system.*

sees and monitors organ procurement and allocation through a nationwide computer system. Canada, Great Britain, and several European countries also have similar organizations to coordinate organ procurement and allocation activities.

An informed public and awareness among health care workers about organ transplantation are necessary for donation to take place. A 1987 Gallup poll showed that 94% of the U.S. public was aware of transplantation and 73% said they would be willing to donate their loved one's organs, if asked.[5] Yet, it is estimated that less than 20% of the potential organ donor pool is realized on an annual basis. As a result of this gap between potential donors and the willingness of the public to donate, 44 states and the District of Columbia have adopted "required request laws."[6] These laws require hospitals to develop procedures for identifying potential organ donors and then informing families of medically suitable candidates about the option to donate their loved one's organs and tissues. Federal legislation was also adopted in

1987 and tied hospital compliance for required request to Medicare reimbursement. Focused educational programs are designed and offered by OPO staff to train health care professionals and keep the public informed about these issues.

Identification, Referral, and Evaluation of the Pediatric Heart Donor

The organ donation process begins when hospital staff identify a patient as a potential organ donor (Fig. 4). Suitable donors have suffered irreversible and total destruction of the brain, are ventilator dependent, and have no history of extracranial malignancies or transmissible diseases (Table 3). Once a potential donor is identified, hospital staff notify a transplant coordinator from the regional OPO. The potential donor's medical suitability is then discussed briefly by telephone.

An on-site evaluation is performed by the transplant coordinator, which includes a thorough review of the patient's history and current medical record. Special laboratory studies are also ordered to assess each organ system being considered for donation. In the case of pediatric heart donors, special attention is given to the assessment of all periods of hypotension, hypoxemia, or arrest, because the pediatric heart is particularly sensitive to the deprivation of oxygen and nutrients. The pediatric patient's need for dopamine or other inotropic support is often an indication of fluid loss and does not necessarily exclude the possibility of heart donation. However, prolonged need for vasopressor support at high dosages (e.g., >20 μg/kg/min dopamine) may indicate underlying cardiac dysfunction or pathology.[7]

This donor assessment information is relayed to the cardiac transplant surgeon, who decides if the heart is suitable for the potential recipient identified (Table 4). The decision to accept a donor heart for transplant is based on (1) normal ECG findings (excluding changes related to CNS insults); (2) a 2-D echocardiogram that shows no structural abnormality, wall-motion disorders, or valvular dysfunction; and (3) an examination by a cardiologist that documents no physical abnormalities. Normal cardiac isoenzymes and arterial blood gases that indicate a pH of 7.35–7.45 and a $P0_2$ of greater than 100 torr provide additional supportive information about suitability.[2]

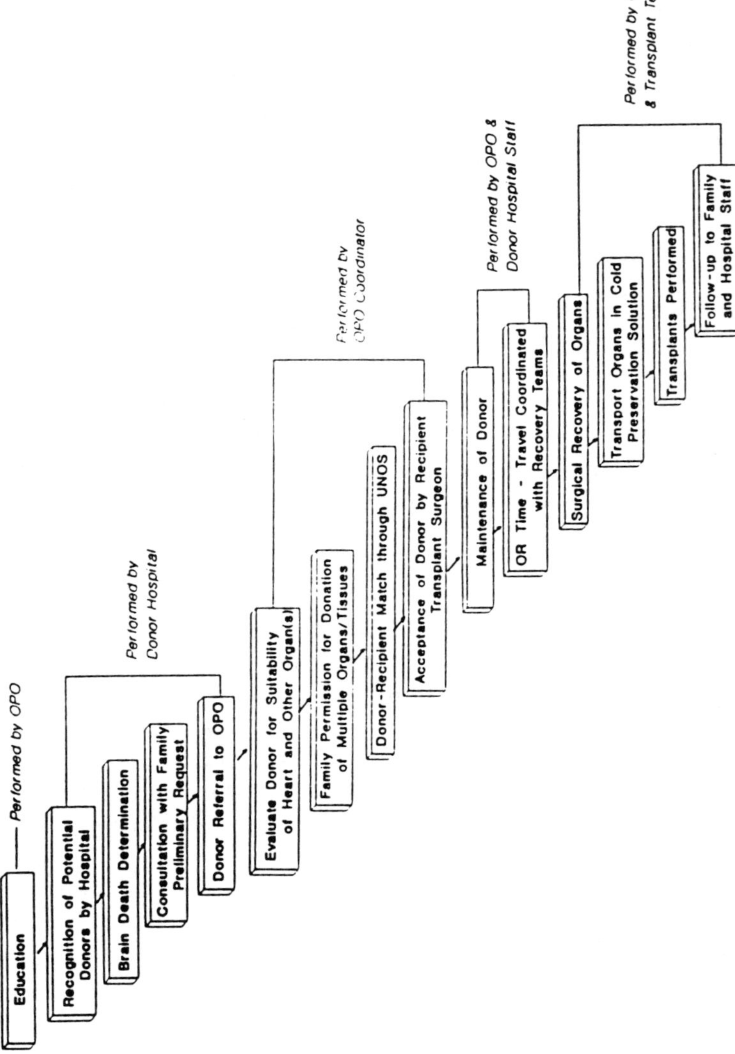

Figure 4: *Steps in organ procurement process.*

Table 3 Contraindications for Organ Donation in the Pediatric Patient

Malignancy, other than primary brain tumor
History of hepatitis or AIDS
Current, untreated bacterial, viral, or fungal septicemia
History of diseases of autoimmune or unknown etiology

Table 4 Potential Donor Assessment Guidelines

INITIAL ASSESSMENT:
Name, age, sex, race
Cause of death
Past medical history
Hospital length of stay
Time on ventilator
Procedures or surgery
Accurate bed weight
Blood pressure trends
Hourly urine output
Medications—vasopressors

TESTS REQUESTED BY OPO:
BUN
Urinalysis
Serum creatinine
Blood type
CBC
ABG
Hepatitis screen
HIV
Serology
Culture reports

ADDITIONAL STUDIES FOR HEART DONATION:
Chest x-ray
12 lead EKG
Cardiology evaluation
2-D echocardiogram (in some cases)
CPK with MB fraction (in some cases)
Description of any cardiac or respiratory arrests

Brain Death

Criteria for the determination of brain death vary nationally and internationally. At present, 44 states have brain death laws, 29 of which have adopted criteria provided by the President's Commission for the Study of Ethical Problems in Medicine and Biomedical and Behavioral Problems (Table 5A).[8] However, the commission expressed caution in the application of this criteria to children under the age of 5 years because the brains of infants and children are more resistant to the effects of hypotension and hypoxemia. This uncertainty in the diagnosis of brain death in infants was described by Coulter. Several infants, who had shown no evidence of clinical brain stem function for periods of up to 48 hours, later recovered with varying degrees of neurologic damage.[9] In light of these occurrences, it is recommended that, in addition to performing clinical examinations to establish brain death in children (Table 5B), at least one confirmatory test be performed. Cerebral angiography, because of its reliability in younger children, is generally considered the confirmatory test of choice. Electroencephalograms (EEG) may be utilized in older children. Declaration of death must be made prior to surgical recovery of organs. It is important to note that the diagnosis of brain death, particularly in the pediatric patient, most often requires a neurospecialist's consultation and should follow the donor institution's brain-death policy.

During the time between brain-death examinations, the potential donor may be evaluated by a transplant coordinator from the regional organ procurement organization to determine suitability and to introduce the subject of organ donation to the family. Close communication between the attending physician, the intensive care unit (ICU) staff,

Table 5A General Criteria for the Determination of Brain Death
Absence of cerebral and brain stem function
Deep coma of irremedial etiology
Persistent absence of all brain function over time
Hypothermia, drug intoxication, metabolic disorders, and shock not present

Table 5B Clinical Tests of Brain Death
Cerebral unresponsiveness
No spontaneous motor activity
Absent pupillary, corneal, and oculocephalic/oculovestibular reflexes
Absent cough reflex with deep tracheal suctioning
No respiratory effort on apnea testing ($PaCO_2$ >60 mm Hg)
Confirmatory test (desirable):
electroencephologram
cerebral blood flow (younger children)

and the transplant coordinator is important so that adequate organ function is maintained during the brain-death evaluation process.

Donor Management

Once brain death has been determined, the emphasis of patient care shifts from interventions protecting the brain to optimizing the stability and function of the vital organs to be donated.[10] Normalizing the pediatric heart donor's blood pressure, oxygenation, urine output, and fluid and electrolyte balance will enhance the suitability of the organs for use in transplantation. Many of the clinical interventions used for this purpose are identical to those chosen to treat a live patient with similar hemodynamic problems. For example, if the donor's hemoglobin is low, transfusion of the appropriate volume of blood will be requested. Likewise, if the donor is losing too much fluid due to diabetes insipidus, dDAVP or Pitressin may be used to decrease urine output.

Treatments often instituted in the care of the pediatric patient being considered as a potential heart donor include[10]:

- Placement of a central line to ensure accurate assessment of hydration and to provide fluid/blood administration accesses.
- Rapid infusion of colloid or Ringer's lactate until satisfactory systolic blood pressure and CVP are obtained.
- Administration of crystalloid to match urine output cc for cc once blood pressure is stabilized.
- If fluid replacement alone does not maintain adequate blood pressure, vasopressor support, preferably low dose dopamine (< 10 μg/kg/min), may be used.
- Close monitoring of electrolytes, with subsequent adjustment of I.V. replacement fluids if patient develops hypernatremia or hypokalemia.
- Ventilator and oxygen adjustments to guarantee $PO_2 \geq 100$.
- Maintenance of sterile technique in wound care, suctioning, etc. It is not uncommon in some situations to cover the patient with prophylactic antibiotics.
- Administration of blood products to maintain hematocrit above 30%.
- Use of warming lights or blankets to maintain body temperature above 34°C.

Generally, organ perfusion is considered to be optimal when urine output is 1–2 cc/kg/hr, blood pressure and CVP are acceptable for donor's age and size, and the PO_2 and oxygenation are acceptable.[10] A donor who is well managed preoperatively in the ICU significantly optimizes not only the potential for a smooth perioperative organ recovery, but also the functioning of the organ in the recipient.

The Donation Request

Approaching a family about organ donation can be a difficult experience for hospital staff because most families are emotionally distraught about their loved one's condition. An important issue to consider prior to introducing the subject of organ donation is the family's acceptance of the diagnosis of brain death. Until the family accepts this diagnosis, the request for donation of organs may be poorly received and most often denied.[11]

The timing of the request may be difficult to judge; however, the period between the clinical examinations to determine brain death may be the most appropriate time to approach a family about organ donation. Because this period often spans at least 12 to 24 hours, the family should have sufficient time to discuss their options.

The Uniform Anatomical Gift Act (UAGA) allows the immediate next of kin to make an anatomical donation of any or all of the decedent's organs and tissues by signing a consent form. In the pediatric donor, the next of kin is usually one or both parents (Table 6).[12] The consent must be witnessed by two individuals and placed on the chart as a permanent part of the patient's record. Families must be assured that only the organs and tissues they have consented to donate will be removed. The OPO transplant coordinators are available to discuss with the family any concerns they may have about donation and to ensure they have given informed consent. Additionally, permission to

Table 6 UAGA Priority Next of Kin

1. Spouse
2. Adult son or daughter
3. Parent
4. Brother or sister
5. Guardian
6. Person charged with disposal of the body

remove organs and tissues must be obtained from the local coroner or medical examiner in circumstances under their jurisdiction.

Organ Allocation

Placement of pediatric donor hearts (and all organs) for transplant is determined by the allocation policies of the United Network for Organ Sharing (UNOS), located in Richmond, Virginia. All waiting recipients are required to be registered with UNOS by a regional organ procurement organization according to certain criteria (Table 7). Once a suitable pediatric donor heart becomes available, certain donor information is entered into the computer by the OPO coordinator to begin recipient matches. The computer identifies a match based on blood type compatibility, donor–recipient size compatibility, length of time on waiting list, urgency of recipient need, and proximity of the donor to the recipient. According to UNOS policy, hearts are allocated first to those pediatric patients found within the service area of the OPO coordinating the recovery process.[13] If no compatible recipients are found within the OPO, then the computer search extends in concentric circles of 500, 1,000, and beyond 1,000 miles. If there is more than one recipient located in a given area, priority is always given to the status 1 recipient. If more than one status 1 recipient is located in a given zone, then the heart will be offered to the pediatric patient who has been waiting the longest. The UNOS computer selects recipients according to blood type–identical donor hearts, unless medical urgency is declared.

Once a potential recipient is identified, the transplant coordinator contacts the responsible transplant surgeon. Based on the information

Table 7 Potential Recipient Information Required for UNOS Computer Listing

Recipient ABO
Recipient age and sex
Acceptable donor weight range
Distance the recipient lives from the transplant center
Recipient status:

Status 1: critical, in ICU, requiring mechanical assist device, ventilator support, or inotropic support
Status 2: stable on medical–surgical floor or waiting at home

presented by the coordinator, the surgeon determines suitability of the heart for that particular recipient. Once a heart is accepted, the surgeon notifies his surgical team, consisting of a surgical assistant, perfusionist, and a transplant coordinator.

Surgical Recovery

Because most pediatric donors have multiple healthy organs, heart removal often occurs concurrently with the removal of kidneys and/or liver. A surgical team for each organ to be retrieved will travel to the donor hospital. In order to properly and successfully retrieve each organ, the surgical teams must work together to simultaneously remove each organ. The organs are flushed and stored in special cold preservation solutions. Hearts are usually arrested with a cardioplegic solution and can be stored no more than 4 hours before circulation must be restored. This short preservation time necessitates precise coordination of the transportation of the organs to the transplant center.

Intraoperative management of the donor is the joint responsibility of the anesthesiologist and the transplant coordinator. Prevention of hypotension, hypoxemia, and acidosis is essential for optimum organ viability. Diuretics are given throughout the procedure to maintain kidney function. Sodium heparin is given immediately prior to the cardioplegic flush and subsequent removal of the heart and other organs.

A multiple organ donor recovery takes approximately 1 to 3 hours intraoperatively. The recipient is prepared for heart implantation as the heart recovery team performs the removal of the heart. Several contacts occur between the donor and recipient teams to limit cold ischemia of the heart. Communications regarding cardiac function and estimated time of arrival with the donor heart are crucial to the transplant team.

When the surgical recovery is completed, the operating room staff and the OPO coordinator provide postmortem care to the donor.

Infant Donor Transport

The recovery of a donor heart from a child less than 6 months of age provides an added challenge to the procurement team. Because the neonatal heart is particularly sensitive to cold ischemia, permission to transport the donor to the recipient institution may be requested to minimize the total time that the heart is without blood flow.

The donor's next of kin must give consent for the transport of their infant. Once this consent is obtained, mobilization of the donor transport team is initiated. This team may include a physician, a nurse, a respiratory therapist, and a transplant coordinator from the OPO. The mode of transportation is determined by the distance between donor and recipient institutions, overall cost of transport, transport time, and availability of appropriate aircraft. This may include a combination of jet aircraft, helicopter, and ambulance.

The transport requires the infant to be placed on 100% O_2 by bagging or by maintaining on portable ventilator, as well as continuance of fluid therapy and appropriate inotropic support. Once the organ recovery is completed, the body is placed in the care of the individual responsible for the transport (usually the transplant coordinator) and returned home.

Anencephalics as Organ Donors

Recent advances in the field of infant heart transplantation have increased the demand for donor organs. In an effort to enlarge the infant donor pool, Loma Linda University Medical Center initiated a protocol designed to support the respiratory and cardiac function of anencephalic infants over a maximum period of 7 days.[12] If the infant fulfilled brain death criteria during this time, organ donation would then be pursued. The protocol was in effect for 7 months during 1988 and was applied to 14 anencephalic infants. Of these 14, only 3 infants fulfilled brain death criteria within the allotted 7-day time period. Only one heart was used for transplantation.[14]

The Loma Linda program was discontinued in July 1988, but the numerous medical and ethical issues surrounding the anencephalic donor remain. Concern still exists over the diagnosis of anencephaly and the wide range of conditions that are termed "anencephaly." Many conditions termed anencephaly may indeed be another neurologic condition. Others questioned whether anencephalics should be subject to the same brain death criteria applied to those who are not "brain absent." Finally, there are concerns directed toward the infants themselves and the justice of carrying them to term for the sole purpose of organ donation. Of the estimated 1,125 anencephalics born each year, it is projected that only 17 hearts would be available and suitable for transplant.[14] These numbers do not reflect the overwhelming potential initially associated with anencephalics as a source for donor hearts.

In the March 1989 issue of *UNOS Update*, an official publication of the National Organ Procurement and Transplantation Network, the UNOS Ethics Committee published its policy regarding the use of organs from anencephalic infants. The committee stated that it is "inappropriate for the anencephalic infant to be subjected to a brain-death determination that is different from that of any other individual." In addition, the committee felt the use of organs from anencephalic infants who did not fulfill brain-death criteria was ill advised.[15]

Summary

The number of pediatric patients waiting for heart transplants continues to grow. The system for recovery and sharing of donor hearts is well organized and sophisticated. Each region of the U.S. and other countries has access to an organ procurement team. However, the major problem related to the procurement of pediatric hearts continues to be the identification of appropriate donors. Because the number of pediatric patients who meet brain-death criteria and fall into the organ donor category is limited, health care professionals must be continually reminded of their responsibility to identify and refer donors to the regional organ procurement organization.

References

1. United Network for Organ Sharing, UNOS Update, June 1988, Vol. 4, Issue 3, p. 6.
2. Bailey NA, Lay P: New horizons: Infant cardiac transplantation. Heart & Lung 1989, 18:172.
3. Kaye MD, Michael P: Registry of the International Society for Heart Transplantation: Sixth Official Report, 1989.
4. Denny D: The Non-physician coordinators' contribution to the development of an organ procurement program. Transplant Proc 1985, 17:83.
5. The US Public's Attitudes Toward Organ Transplants/Organ Donation. The Gallup Organization, Princeton, NJ, 1987.
6. Evaluation of Methods Used by States to Expand the Number of Organ and Tissue Donors, (HRSA Contract #240-86-0048). Maximus, Inc., 1988.

7. North American Transplant Coordinators (NATCO), An Introductory Course on Procurement for Transplant Coordinators, May 1987.
8. Guidelines for the determination of death: Medical consultants on the diagnosis of death to the President's Commission for the Study of Ethical Problems in Medicine and Biomedical and Behavioral Research. JAMA 1981, 246:2184.
9. Coulter DL: Neurologic uncertainty in newborn intensive care. N Engl J Med 1987, 316:840.
10. Darby JM, Stein K, Grenvik A, et al: Approach to management of the heartbeating "brain dead" organ donor. JAMA 1989, 261:2222.
11. Howard S: "How do I ask?" Nursing 89:70.
12. Lee P, Kessner P: Organ donation and the uniform anatomical gift act. Surgery 1986, 100:867.
13. United Network for Organ Sharing Policy Manual, Policy on Heart and Heart/Lung Allocation, Policy #3.7, December 6, 1988, pp. 9–12.
14. Shewmon DA, et al: The use of anencephalic infants as organ sources. JAMA 1989, 261:1773.
15. United Network for Organ Sharing, UNOS Update, March 1989, Special Edition; Vol. 5, Issue 3.

Chapter 5

Anesthetic Considerations in Pediatric Cardiac Transplantation

David A. Lowe

Introduction

The major issues of concern to the anesthesiologist caring for a child undergoing cardiac transplantation are:

1. *Protection of the donor heart* until it is harvested
2. *Prebypass management of the recipient* with end-stage heart disease, who has little or no cardiac reserve, yet extreme cardiovascular sensitivity to noxious stimulation, anesthetic drugs, and operative manipulation
3. *Weaning the donor heart from bypass,* a heart that is permanently denervated and temporarily ischemic, yet required for the first time to eject against an increased, sometimes overwhelming, pulmonary vascular resistance (PVR)
4. *Concern for infection* throughout each of these phases because control of infection may require reduction or elimination of immunosuppressive drugs

Management of the Donor

Before Determination of Brain Death

The donor heart begins as an innocent bystander that is threatened by: (1) the loss of neurologic function, (2) the therapeutic inter-

From *Heart Transplantation in Children,* edited by Jeffrey M. Dunn, M.D. and Richard M. Donner, M.D.

vention designed to decrease intracranial pressure, (3) infection, and sometimes (4) a reduction in care around the time of the determination of brain death. Although the responsibility of the donor hospital, it is essential for the transplant team to coordinate and direct the management of the donor to assure a healthy organ.

Hemodynamic instability is inevitable with the loss of sympathetic tone that occurs with severe neurologic injury.[1] The systemic vascular resistance (SVR) is reduced, the venous capacitance is increased, and the compensatory mechanisms that ordinarily preserve the central circulation are eliminated. Peripheral vasodilatation prevents the body from conserving heat and combines with the loss of central thermoregulatory control to make hypothermia likely. The intravascular volume becomes vulnerable when an excessive volume of extremely dilute urine is produced as occurs in about 50% of donors as a result of central diabetes insipidus and in another 25% from some other cause, such as the high output phase of acute tubular necrosis or the osmotic diuretic effect of hyperglycemia, mannitol, or contrast media. For patients with central diabetes insipidus, intravenous infusion of aqueous vasopressin simplifies fluid management and minimizes the risk of wide fluid and electrolyte shifts. The starting dose, 100 μU/kg/hr, produces blood levels within the physiologic range. This rate is doubled every 15–30 min until the urine output is reduced to 2–4 mL/kg/hr and the urine osmolality is raised to at least twice that of the plasma.[2] The effectiveness of desmopressin (dDAVP) has been impressive in a dose of 5–20 μg intranasally or one-tenth this dose intravenously as a bolus. Although the biologic half-life of desmopressin is variable and usually needs to be repeated every 12 hours, it avoids the significant vasoconstrictive effect produced by the higher rates of vasopressin infusion.[3]

Hemodynamic instability is further assured by efforts to decrease the intracranial pressure. Deliberate fluid restriction, diuretic therapy, and osmotherapy aiming for a serum osmolarity of 300–320 mOsm are designed to produce a preload that is, at best, marginal and often so low as to require inotropic support to maintain a cardiac output that is just barely adequate. Deliberate hyperventilation leads to alkalemia, hypokalemia, and a low ionized calcium. Frequently, thiopental in 1–2-mg/kg boluses and/or lidocaine in 1–1.5-mg/kg boluses are administered to treat spikes in intracranial pressure or to prevent spikes prior to noxious stimulation, such as with endotracheal tube suctioning and chest physiotherapy. Sustained intracranial pressures over 20 mmHg may be treated with deliberate hypothermia (34°–35°C) and pentobarbital coma, both decreasing the state of myocardial contractility. Ventricular fibrillation may be precipitated by the combination of hypothermia and hypokalemia.

Potential organ donors also have an increased risk of infection. Bacteria may have been introduced at the time of the injury or perhaps during vascular access at the time of the resuscitation, when sterile technique was a low priority. Hypothermia depresses immunocompetence, and any low cardiac output state, reducing splanchnic blood flow, predisposes to bacterial invasion from the gut. Pneumonia is more likely because aggressive chest percussion and postural drainage are often withheld in patients with increased intracranial pressure, even those who presented having aspirated blood or vomitus.

After Determination of Brain Death

At the time of the determination of brain death, the priorities are shifted to protect the donor heart and its life-support system. The intravascular volume is aggressively restored, usually eliminating the need for inotropic support.[4] Diuretic therapy and osmotherapy are no longer indicated. The ventilatory settings are adjusted to achieve normocarbia and optimal PEEP, while aggressive chest physiotherapy is established to provide thorough tracheobronchial toilet. Normothermia is achieved by warming the inspired gases to 37°C with 100% humidification, the intravenous fluids to 37°C (including crystalloid), and the body surface with a circulating water mattress and overhead radiant warmer lamps. The donor heart is further protected by prophylactic antibiotics and by replacement of contaminated catheters.

The beneficial effect of triiodothyronine (T_3) for the brain-dead potential organ donor is of considerable interest, but awaits controlled trials. Novitsky and Cooper[5] observed increasing anaerobic metabolism and lactic acidosis in brain-dead donors associated with diminishing myocardial function. They then observed increasing aerobic metabolism and improving myocardial function while 2 μg of triiodothyronine were administered each hour from the determination of brain-death until the excision of the heart. They concluded that this improvement enabled them to salvage some donor hearts that would otherwise have been unusable and to transplant all hearts in as good a condition as possible.

Because of the ongoing threat of cardiovascular instability, the brain-dead donor requires the same standard of care that the anesthesiologist would provide to any critically ill patient during transport and during the harvesting procedure.[6] Essential intraoperative monitoring includes the esophageal stethoscope and temperature probe, ECG, noninvasive blood pressure, pulse oximetry, end-tidal CO_2, and urine output. Central venous pressure monitoring is also essential; intra-arterial pressure monitoring is often helpful. A pulmonary artery (PA) catheter is never necessary when a healthy heart is being harvested.

The anesthesiologist must be prepared to promptly administer large volumes of crystalloid and blood products through at least one short, large-bore, intravenous catheter. When systemic hypotension persists despite a CVP as high as 10–12 mmHg, a low SVR can be increased with an alpha agonist, such as phenylephrine in boluses of 1–10 μg/kg or by constant infusion in doses of 0.1–1.0 μg/kg/min. Some inotropic support with dopamine up to 10 μg/kg/min may be necessary due to the ablation of normal autonomic responses.[7] When harvesting includes the kidneys and liver, vasoconstrictors are relatively contraindicated, although a vasoconstrictor that increases the renal perfusion pressure when the SVR is very low can improve renal blood flow and glomerular filtration, as verified by an increase in urine output. The margin of safety will be increased by delivering 100% oxygen and by maintaining the hematocrit between 30% and 40% in patients whose blood has been diluted with crystalloid. A rise in hematocrit will increase the blood viscosity and thereby the SVR, helping to insure an adequate perfusion pressure in addition to improving oxygen- carrying capacity.

Although anesthetic agents are unnecessary, blood pressure and heart rate may increase in brain-dead patients in response to surgical stimulation.[8] A nondepolarizing muscle relaxant will improve surgical exposure when residual muscle tone exists. The donor undergoes anticoagulation with 300 units/kg of beef-lung heparin prior to organ removal.[9] When the kidneys are to be harvested, intravenous phentolamine (0.1 mg/kg) maximizes dilatation and prevents spasm of the renal arteries.[10,11] The bolus of phentolamine is administered when the surgeon is prepared to selectively perfuse the organs, moments after profound hypotension signals the effect of this potent α-adrenergic receptor blocker.

Management of the Recipient

Pathophysiology and Hemodynamic Objectives

Any child with end-stage heart disease who survives to reach the operating room has little or no cardiovascular reserve, yet extreme cardiovascular sensitivity to anesthetic agents, noxious stimuli, and operative manipulation. This applies to a child with compensated congestive failure on modest medical therapy who arrives breathing room air and certainly to a child with a barely viable cardiac output despite dobutamine, dopamine, amrinone, nitroprusside, lidocaine, an intra-aortic balloon pump, and mechanical ventilation.

Pathophysiology and hemodynamic objectives concern heart rate, preload, contractility, and afterload.

Heart Rate

The failing ventricle in a patient with end-stage dilated cardiomyopathy produces a critically reduced stroke volume because of the combined effects of poor myocardial contractility and the mechanical burden of the dilated heart.[12] Therefore, maintenance of a sinus rhythm at a normal to a high-normal rate is critically important. Even the loss of the atrial kick with a nodal rhythm can be devastating in a patient at risk for more serious dysrhythmias from any of the following causes: the primary disease, myocardial ischemia, atrial distension, vagal stimulation with airway manipulation, the undesired chronotropic effect of inotropes, the release of endogenous catecholamines with noxious stimulation during light anesthesia, hypercarbia, mechanical stimulation by an intracardiac wire during insertion of a central venous catheter, mechanical stimulation by the surgeon, hypokalemia, hypothermia, and digitalis toxicity.

Preload

Whether the patient has an intracardiac tumor or pericardial disease limiting end-diastolic volume, or a primary cardiomyopathy associated with a huge end-diastolic volume, each patient will have an optimal end-diastolic volume with very little tolerance for hypervolemia or hypovolemia. Unlike the normal patient, in whom increases in end-diastolic volume produce increases in stroke volume, the Frank-Starling curve of the dilated heart is flattened and displaced downward and to the right, describing how a small increase in end-diastolic volume will produce little, if any, increase in stroke volume.[13,14] This occurs because the sarcomere length is at or near its functional upper limit so that contraction, which depends on the overlap of actin and myosin fibrils, is much less responsive to increases in preload.[15] Conversely, a small decrease in preload may have a dramatic effect because any further decrease in stroke volume initiates the vicious cycle of cardiogenic failure leading to multisystem organ failure and lactic acidosis further reducing pump function.

The anesthesiologist is responsible for identifying and preserving the optimal preload when the patient is likely to experience reductions in absolute blood volume as well as reductions in effective blood volume by drugs with vasodilating effects (particularly venodilators), positive pressure ventilation that impedes venous return, and such surgical manipulations as the creation of the pericardial cradle, direct compression of the heart, and venous cannulation.

Contractility

There can also be no further decrease in the state of contractility. Not only will the myocardial depressant effect of ischemia, many of the anesthetic agents, an abnormal pH, hypothermia, and hypocalcemia be poorly tolerated, but inotropic agents cannot be relied upon to improve stroke volume. After chronic exposure to excessive catecholamine levels,[16] adrenergic mechanisms that modulate the heart's inotropic state become less sensitive to β_1 adrenergic stimulation because of a reduction in the density and sensitivity of β_1 receptors.[17,18] Receptor uncoupling (a physical separation of the receptor subunit from the regulatory subunit that activates the adenylate cyclase enzyme) and receptor down-regulation (a process whereby fewer membrane receptors are available for activation as the β-receptor subunit becomes engulfed within the cytoplasm) occur in proportion to the degree and duration of clinical heart failure. These receptor defects account for the diminished effectiveness of drugs that act directly to stimulate the β-adrenergic receptor, often requiring higher than ordinary doses of epinephrine, isoproterenol, norepinephrine, dopamine, and dobutamine, as well as the relative effectiveness of drugs that do not rely on the β_1 receptor, such as the β_2 agonists, α_1 myocardial agonists, digitalis, glucagon, and the phosphodiesterase inhibitors, such as amrinone.[19–21]

Afterload

As predicted by Laplace's law, the work of the failing heart is already increased by the high intraventricular systolic pressures needed to overcome pulmonary and systemic vasoconstriction, as well as by the elevations in end-diastolic volume as myocardial function worsens.[22] Unlike the normal heart, in which the wall stress decreases precipitously with ejection as the ventricular radius decreases and wall thickness increases, the wall stress in the dilated heart is elevated at the beginning of systole and rises during early systole because of the relatively small decrease in ventricular volume and the insignificant increase in wall thickness.[12,23] This inability of the dilated heart to unload itself during systole, combined with its poor contractility, results in a much greater decrease in stroke volume for any increase in afterload, as compared to the normal heart that would experience only a slight decrease in stroke volume with a comparable increase in afterload.[24]

Further increases in right ventricular afterload are likely to be precipitated by a low alveolar oxygen concentration, hypoxemia, acidemia (respiratory or metabolic), hypothermia, elevated or reduced functional residual capacity, straining and crying, increased α-adrenergic tone, polycythemia, increased right ventricular preload, left ventricular failure, very negative pleural pressure, and, possibly, nitrous oxide. (Table 1).[25–28] Children with increased PA pressures are especially sensitive to these precipitants and are in greater jeopardy of having periodic, dramatic, and sometimes lethal increases in their PVR causing right ventricular failure.

The anesthesiologist's objective is to avoid these precipitating factors and to promote pulmonary vasodilatation. In severe cases, this would include delivery of 100% oxygen, profound general anesthesia, the establishment of both a metabolic and respiratory alkalosis, mechanical ventilation with optimal, not excessive, PEEP, and paralysis.

Table 1 Further Increases in Right Ventricular Afterload

Alveolar hypoxia
Hypoxemia
Acidemia (respiratory or metabolic)
Hypothermia
Elevated or reduced functional residual capacity
Straining/crying
Increased α-adrenergic tone
Polycythemia
Increased right ventricular preload
Left ventricular failure
Very negative pleural pressure
? Nitrous oxide

In addition, inotropes, arteriodilators and venodilators, and perhaps an intra-aortic balloon pump will be necessary to further reduce the transpulmonary pressure gradient (mean PA pressure minus pulmonary capillary wedge pressure) and to maintain an adequate cardiac output and coronary perfusion pressure. In a patient with a marginal circulation, another fundamental objective is to prevent the increases in metabolic demand that occur with pain and anxiety, light anesthesia, hyperthermia, hypothermia and shivering.

Pulmonary vasodilatation is not desirable in neonates with hypoplastic left heart syndrome in whom a single ventricle is ejecting into two parallel circulations that are competing for the available cardiac output. Pulmonary vasodilatation would increase the pulmonary blood flow and the oxygen content of the blood. However, because this would occur at the expense of the systemic and coronary blood flow that depends upon a patent ductus arteriosus, the oxygen delivery to the tissues would be substantially reduced.[29] Instead, optimal oxygen delivery to the tissues is more likely to result from a balanced circulation. Excessive pulmonary blood flow can be avoided by maintaining a normal PCO_2 and by restricting the FiO_2, at least until the PaO_2 reaches 90 mmHg. Some patients may benefit by reducing the FiO_2 until the PaO_2 reaches 40 mmHg when the arterial saturation is slightly over 80%, just at the beginning of the plateau of the newborn's fetal oxygen–hemoglobin dissociation curve. Also, pharmacologic pulmonary vasodilators must be used cautiously, including prostaglandin E_1, which is continued by constant infusion to inhibit closure of the patent ductus arteriosus until cardiopulmonary bypass.

Preoperative Evaluation and Preparation

Any child selected for cardiac transplantation will have severe functional impairment and secondary compromise of renal, hepatic, and pulmonary function that is expected to be reversed by a higher cardiac output and lower systemic and pulmonary venous pressures.[30–32] Preoperatively, the anesthesiologist must become familiar with the patient's current cardiovascular function and the support required to optimize it. A set of realistic hemodynamic objectives must be determined for each patient, with the assumption that little or no variation will be tolerated, whether the patient is ambulatory or bedridden, normotensive and well perfused, or hypotensive and acidotic. The preoperative anesthetic evaluation provides an opportunity for the anesthesiologist to earn the trust of the parents and then the child.

Premedication with sedatives and analgesics is relatively contraindicated and usually withheld. Sedatives and analgesics may take away any remaining ability the child has to compensate for the low cardiac output state and they may reduce the value of the mental status examination in the assessment of the adequacy of the central circulation. However, most patients who are old enough to be concerned about the risk of the procedure are also sophisticated enough about their disease to realize its purpose. They are likely to be calmed by a gentle approach and the reassurance that they will be either sedated or induced with general anesthesia soon after arriving in the operating room.

The preoperative evaluation and remaining preparation of the patient, preparation of the anesthesia supplies and equipment in the operating room, transport to the operating room, and the induction of anesthesia before or after the insertion of invasive catheters must be performed early enough to guarantee that the surgeon can place the patient on bypass at the time of the arrival of the donor heart to prevent prolongation of the donor heart's ischemic time. The need to protect the donor heart by limiting ischemic time also justifies proceeding when a patient has had an inadequate period of preoperative starvation. As long as the oral preoperative dose of cyclosporine is not mixed with food or milk to make it more palatable, even the maximum dose of 5 mg/kg is not enough to generate concern for a "full stomach" because a 20-kg child would only receive a volume of 1 mL.

Preparation of the anesthesia equipment must be completed before the patient arrives in the operating room in order to monitor the patient without distraction and to respond immediately to expected and unexpected problems. Although the preparation for airway management, fluid administration, monitoring, temperature control, and the administration of anesthesia is relatively straightforward, there is wide institutional variability concerning the setup of nonanesthetic drugs. The resuscitative and vasoactive drugs prepared in advance at our institution are listed in Table 2. All bolus drugs are drawn up in an appropriate sized syringe with the air bubbles evacuated and the label clearly marked. In every case, at least four vasoactive drugs for constant infusion are prepared in advance (epinephrine, isoproterenol, dopamine, and nitroprusside) based on formulations that are easy to manage, easy to remember, and provide a reasonable amount of fluid infused within the normal dose range. By putting 0.6 mg/kg of epinephrine in D_5W to total 100 mL, 1 mL/hr will be equal to the starting dose of 0.1 µg/kg/min. The same formulation applies to isoproterenol

Table 2 Nonanesthetic Drugs Routinely Prepared in Advance

	Dose	Syringe
	Resuscitative Drugs by Bolus	
Atropine	0.2 mg/kg (max 0.4 mg)	0.4 mg/mL in 3 mL
Epinephrine	1–10 µg/kg	1 µg/kg/mL in 10 mL
Isoproterenol	1–10 µg/kg	1 µg/kg/mL in 10 mL
Bicarbonate	.5–1 mEq/kg	1 mEq/mL in 20 mL
infants ≤ 6 mos		.5 mEq/mL in 20 mL
Lidocaine 1%	1 mg/kg	10 mg/mL in 10 mL
Phenylephrine	3–10 µg/kg	100 µg/mL in 10 mL
Calcium gluconate 10%	10–30 mg/kg peripherally	100 mg/mL in 10 mL
Calcium chloride 10%	3–10 mg/kg centrally	100 mg/mL in 10 mL
	Vasoactive Drugs by Constant Infusion	
Isoproterenol	0.1–1.0 µg/kg/min	0.6 mg/kg in 100 mL
Epinephrine	0.1–1.0 µg/kg/min	1 mL/hr = 0.1 µg/kg/min
*Norepinephrine	0.1–1.0 µg/kg/min	
Dopamine	5–10 µg/kg/min	6 mg/kg in 100 mL
*Dobutamine	5–10 µg/kg/min	1 mL/hr = 1 µg/kg/min
*Amrinone (after 0.75 mg/kg bolus)	5–10 µg/kg/min	
Nitroprusside	1–5 µg/kg/min	
*Nitroglycerin	1–5 µg/kg/min	
*Prostaglandin E_1	30–150 ng/kg/min	500 µg in 50 mL 0.6 mL × kg = 100 ng/kg/min

*Prepared only when specifically indicated.

and norepinephrine. Placing 6 mg/kg of dopamine, dobutamine, amrinone, nitroprusside, or nitroglycerin in a total of 100 mL will result in 1 mL/hr delivering 1 μg/kg/min. When one 500-μg ampule of PGE_1 is placed in 50 mL of D_5W, a rate equal to 0.6 mL times the weight in kilograms will deliver 100 ng/kg/min.

Just prior to transport, the proper position of all tubes and catheters is verified, secured, and organized. Specific personnel must be assigned to the physical tasks involved in transport so that others can be devoted to monitoring the patient and providing respiratory and cardiovascular support.

Intraoperative Monitoring and Vascular Access

Once the patient is transferred to the operating table without displacing tubes and catheters or causing the patient to exert himself, the precordial stethoscope, ECG, pulse oximeter probe, noninvasive blood pressure cuff, and axillary temperature probe are applied, and any supplemental oxygen that the patient was receiving is maintained. After the child is intubated, continuous end-tidal CO_2, nasopharyngeal temperature, and urinary output monitoring are established.

All tubes and catheters are inserted with meticulous aseptic technique. It is realistic to assume that any violation in technique may introduce infection that becomes evident only days after the anesthesiologist had been involved, requiring immunosuppressants to be weaned and perhaps leading to rejection of the donor heart.

Peripheral venous or femoral venous access is required before proceeding to the induction of general anesthesia or the placement of other invasive monitors. Invasive monitors are inserted prior to induction whenever the patient's ability to cooperate, intravenous sedation, and local anesthesia combine to make the procedure feasible and acceptable. Percutaneous radial or femoral arterial catheterization can be accomplished without upsetting the child if 1–3 mL of 0.5% lidocaine ($\leq$2 mg/kg) without epinephrine are delivered subcutaneously and the infiltration that results is eliminated over 15 min by intermittent compression.

Percutaneous internal jugular vein cannulation requires substantially more cooperation and/or intravenous sedation because the child's face must be partially covered by sterile towels and since orthopnea may occur in the supine position. The high systemic venous pressure makes cannulation relatively easy and the Trendelenburg position unnecessary. If aseptic technique cannot be maintained, or if the child becomes unresponsive to voice after incremental doses of intravenous midazolam (0.03 mg/kg) while oxygen is delivered under the drapes, the procedure is postponed until after the induction of anesthesia when ventilation is controlled. The right internal jugular vein remains the preferred route for central venous access in children, whereas the left internal jugular vein is used in adults so that the right internal jugular can be cannulated repetitively by the cardiologist who performs serial transvenous endomyocardial biopsies to determine the presence or degree of graft rejection over the long term.[33]

The guidelines used in our institution for the selection of pulmonary artery catheters in children are indicated in Table 3. For children up to 1 year of age, who usually weigh less than 10 kg, a 5F, 5-cm, double-lumen catheter is inserted into the right internal jugular vein and cardiac output is measured with a 2F, no-lumen, thermistor catheter introduced into the main PA through the right ventricular wall by the surgeon prior to coming off bypass.[34] For children between 1 and 2 years of age, who weigh 10–13 kg, a 5F, thermodilution, PA catheter is inserted with the proximal lumen 10 cm from the distal port. In children between 3 and 6 years of age, who weigh 15–20 kg, the proximal lumen is 15 cm from the distal port. In children between 7 and 14 years of age, who weigh 25–50 kg, a 7F, thermodilution catheter with a proximal lumen 20 cm from the end is used, and in children over 14 years, who generally weigh over 50 kg, a 7F catheter with a proximal lumen 30 cm from the tip is inserted. The 5F and 7F catheters are chosen with the goal of having the proximal lumen in the right atrium separated from the PA by two valves. Our estimates of the distance in centimeters from the midatrial position of the central venous port to the wedge position are somewhat greater than those predicted by the equation: $5.32 + 1.06 \times$ square root of age in months, as determined by a study on 40 cadavers (with empty hearts)

Table 3 Guidelines for Selection of Pulmonary Artery Catheters

Age	Weight (kg)	French	Proximal Lumen (cm)
< 1 yr	< 10	2	
1–2 yr	10–13	5	10
3–6 yr	15–20	5	15
7–14 yr	25–50	7	20
> 14 yr	> 50	7	30

and 20 children undergoing cardiac catheterization in whom there was no mention of heart size.[35]

A rapid-response, thermistor, PA catheter is now available for adult-sized patients with pulmonary hypertension and right ventricular dysfunction.[36] Unlike the thermistor response of the standard, thermistor-tipped, PA catheter that is 300–1,000 msec, the response time of this catheter is reduced to 50 msec, so that beat-to-beat variations in temperature are seen on a thermodilution cardiac output curve. The measurement of temperature changes associated with successive diastolic plateaus permits the computation of an average right ventricular ejection fraction over 4–5 beats, in addition to the determination of cardiac output, right ventricular end-diastolic volume, systolic volume, and stroke volume. Oximetry catheters for continuous measurement of mixed venous oxygen saturations are not used routinely at our institution.

Some anesthesiologists, including the author, believe that a PA catheter is indicated for every cardiac transplant recipient, including those who are not considered to have pulmonary hypertension.[37] This approach is justified either by removing the catheter within 24–72 hours of insertion before the risk of catheter-related infections becomes excessive[38] or by replacing it with another through a different insertion site. If the PA catheter does not float easily into the PA because of the low flow within the enlarged heart, or if arrhythmias are precipitated, the catheter is maintained within a sterile sleeve attached to the introducer with its tip in the superior vena cava to be advanced later, manually, by the surgeon into the new heart. This sterile sleeve protects the catheter exiting from the introducer and allows catheter repositioning following initial placement because the external catheter remains sterile for 1.7 ± 0.2 days after insertion, despite to-and-fro manipulation during cardiopulmonary bypass.[39] Left atrial lines are placed by the surgeon in all patients, including neonates, eliminating the need for a PA-occluded pressure and increasing the accuracy of assessing left-sided pressure.

Induction and Maintenance of Anesthesia

Throughout the induction of anesthesia, the anesthesiologist allows for an increased circulation time because patients with a low cardiac output and a decreased ejection fraction have delayed, often exaggerated, responses to drugs with cardiovascular effects.[12,40] Dramatic effects will be even more likely if the initial volume of distribution is reduced by peripheral vasoconstriction and/or hypovolemia as a greater amount of the drug is delivered to the cerebral and coronary circulation. So, in these patients with little or no cardiovascular reserve, but with a normal anesthetic requirement, a very slow induction is performed with small incremental doses until the cumulative dosage meets their anesthetic requirement.[41]

The most popular induction technique is to administer 100% oxygen while delivering small incremental doses until a total of 50–100 μg/kg of fentanyl or 10–30 μg/kg of sufentanil has been administered prior to the incision.[42] Such a high-dose narcotic technique provides acceptable, intraoperative, hemodynamic stability for most patients with blunting of the neuroendocrine response accompanying intubation, skin incision, and sternotomy.[43–49] Although narcotics are often chosen because of their minimal depressant effects on cardiovascular function, hypotension may occur as the patient goes to sleep with loss of sympathetic tone, requiring volume expansion, perhaps an increase in inotropic support, and sometimes even pharmacologic restoration of α-adrenergic tone.

The narcotic is titrated (for example, fentanyl, 1 μg/kg each minute for 5 min, followed by larger increments) as various stimuli of increasing magnitude are introduced, such as the application of a tourniquet, the performance of a jaw thrust, the insertion of an oral airway, laryngoscopy, and endotracheal intubation.[50] The goal is for the anesthesiologist to assess the depth of anesthesia following each stimulus to determine the dose of narcotic necessary to maintain an adequate depth of anesthesia with subsequent stimuli, while gradually reducing what may be a high resting sympathetic tone that maintains the patient's hemodynamic state. Inadequate anesthesia may not be reflected by a rise in blood pressure. Instead, the blood pressure may stay the same or decrease as the surge of endogenous catecholamines causes even more intense pulmonary and systemic vasoconstriction and perhaps triggers dysrhythmias.[51]

Early on, respiratory depression by the narcotic will need to be offset by assisted, then controlled, ventilation. Once effective positive pressure ventilation has been demonstrated, the patient is paralyzed with a nondepolarizing muscle relaxant and intubation is performed, usually after 10%–50% of the total narcotic has been administered. The muscle relaxant may be indicated earlier if the narcotic induces chest-wall rigidity, although this will be less likely the more slowly the narcotic is administered. The increased vagal tone produced by the narcotic will cause slowing of the heart rate, a problem in a patient who is dependent on a resting tachycardia. This problem can be prevented by the prophylactic use of atropine and the selection of pancuronium for its vagolytic effect.

Increments of diazepam (0.1 mg/kg) or midazolam (0.03 mg/kg) are often added to produce hypnotic and amnestic effects while blunting the catecholamine responses sometimes encountered during a pure narcotic anesthetic.[42] They must be used with great caution, however, because the combination of a narcotic and a benzodiazepine causes hypotension as a result of vasodilatation and, in larger does, a decrease in contractility.[48,52–56] Scopolamine (0.02 mg/kg with a maximum of 0.4 mg) is an alternative to prevent awareness without effecting myocardial contractility.

Barbituates and potent inhalation agents, such as halothane and isoflurane, are myocardial depressants and are relatively contraindicated as primary anesthetics in patients with poor ventricular function, although thiopental and halothane were used in the first successful human heart transplant in 1967.[57] Since then, the incidence of precardiopulmonary bypass hypotension has been significantly greater in patients anesthetized with volatile anesthetics as compared to patients who received narcotics.[12,42,51]

It is not uncommon for a cardiac transplant recipient to arrive with what is assumed to be a "full stomach" and risk of aspiration, although there is usually sufficient notice to arrange for the patient to be NPO long enough for the stomach to empty prior to induction. Each of the alternatives described below can reduce the risk of aspiration, while preserving hemodynamic stability in patients with severe ventricular dysfunction and a full stomach provided the anesthesiologist effectively gains control of the patient's airway.

A rapid-sequence induction and intubation consisting of preoxygenation, cricoid pressure, ketamine (1 mg/kg), and succinylcholine (1.5–2 mg/kg) has provided a record of safety.[42,58] Because the prevention of aspiration depends upon a rapid onset of effect, these drugs should be delivered centrally when a central venous or PA catheter is in place. Ketamine ordinarily increases blood pressure and heart rate because it provokes the release of endogenous catecholamines that obscure its mild direct negative inotropic effect.[59,60] However, the possibility of some cardiac depression from ketamine must be anticipated in patients with severe heart failure in whom β-receptor down-regulation, receptor uncoupling, and myocardial catecholamine depletion come to render the patient unresponsive to the sympathetic effects of ketamine. Although ketamine was initially considered to increase PVR in patients with pulmonary vascular disease,[61,62] more recent studies in pediatric patients with both normal and elevated PVR have shown no increase in PVR when the PCO_2 and PaO_2 were maintained within the normal ranges.[63,64]

Another option is to provide preoxygenation, cricoid pressure, and fentanyl (10 μg/kg), etomidate (0.3 mg/kg), and succinylcholine (1.5 mg/kg) in rapid-sequence fashion. Following induction, anesthesia is maintained with careful titration of fentanyl until 50–100 μg/kg is administered prior to sternotomy. This technique has been reported to provide hemodynamic stability with minimal response to intubation in adult cardiac transplant recipients with severe ventricular dysfunction (ejection fractions ≤20%) and full stomachs.[65]

A modified rapid-sequence technique, providing a more gentle induction that still minimizes the risk of vomiting and regurgitation, can be achieved with preoxygenation, the continuous application of cricoid pressure, and 15–30 μg/kg of fentanyl[66,67] or 5–10 μg/kg of sufentanil,[68] both immediately, followed by pancuronium (0.15 mg/kg) with gentle, controlled ventilation by bag and mask until endotracheal intubation 90 sec later.

Nitrous oxide is not used as an adjunct to maintain anesthesia during cardiac transplantation. It will increase the size of any air emboli and decrease the inspired oxygen concentration. One hundred percent oxygen is a pulmonary vasodilator, it helps protect the patient from hypoxemia due to hypoventilation and intrapulmonary shunting, and it also minimizes the size of any obvious or occult air emboli. There is also some concern about nitrous oxide acting as a mild myocardial depressant[69–71] and perhaps increasing the PVR in children. Studies in adults have consistently documented that nitrous oxide increases PVR, causing small increases in patients with normal PVR and large increases in patients with pulmonary hypertension.[72,73] These findings in adults, however, were not observed in the only comparable study in infants.[74]

Cardiopulmonary Bypass

Cardiopulmonary bypass, which is initiated either just before or upon the arrival of the donor heart, is managed in the ordinary fashion with flow rates of 2.5 L/M^2 when the body temperature is normal and at half these flow rates when the body temperature is taken to 24°–26°C, except in the newborn who is taken to 17°–18°C prior to total circulatory arrest. A long period of rewarming is necessary because of the prolonged ischemic time. Just prior to removal of the aortic cross clamp, the patient is placed in a head-down position to reduce the risk of cerebral air emboli should any air remain in the heart. Methylprednisolone (10 mg/kg) is administered when the new heart is perfused for the first time, and ATG (10 mg/kg/hr × 4 hr) is begun once bypass is terminated.

Postbypass Management of the Donor Heart and Pulmonary Hypertension

Physiology of the Transplanted Heart

Weaning the transplanted heart from bypass begins with an understanding of these fundamental problems: (1) the denervation that is complete and permanent; (2) the global ischemia that occurs despite optimal myocardial preservation technique, accounting for a relatively fixed stroke volume and a relatively rate-dependent cardiac output until the heart recovers to demonstrate normal contractility and a normal Frank-Starling effect; and (3) the susceptibility of the right ventricle to an increased, sometimes overwhelming, PVR that is capable of exaggerated responses to ordinary stimulants of pulmonary vasoconstriction.

Denervation

Complete and permanent denervation of the transplanted heart produces an ECG that looks strange even in the best of circumstances. The ECG reveals two P waves, one produced by the recipient's sinus node that remains innervated and the other produced by the donor's sinus node that has been denervated and remains denervated for the duration of the recipient's life.[75] These P waves are totally independent of one another, with the donor heart rate a little faster than that of the recipient, probably because of the loss of autonomic tone that is predominantly parasympathetic.[76] Free from resting vagal tone, the chronically transplanted heart has a resting rate of 90–120 beats/min in the adult. The recipient's sinus node rate remains responsive to neural impulses transmitted to this remnant of right atrial tissue, but only those P waves produced by the donor atrial tissue are conducted, just as they would be in the innervated heart.[77]

Another major characteristic of the denervated heart is its response to physiologic and pharmacologic manipulations. For example, without the baroreceptor reflex, the denervated heart lacks the ability to respond acutely with tachycardia to raise the cardiac output when the systemic blood pressure falls because of hypovolemia, vasodilatation, or decreased myocardial contractility. Similarly, the disruption of autonomic neurotransmission prevents immediate responses in donor heart rate and contractility to pain, anxiety, and noxious stimulation under light anesthesia. The donor heart rate will increase, but only when circulating catecholamines increase.[78,79] Until then, the transplant recipient is vulnerable to insults that require a rapid increase in heart rate and contractility, such as a decrease in venous return, a decrease in vascular resistance, or a sudden increase in metabolic demand. Intravascular volume depletion is poorly tolerated, particularly when anesthetic agents, such as halothane and isoflurane, suppress the sympathoadrenal system or vasodilators defeat the sympathoadrenal system.

The denervated heart only responds to vasoactive drugs that have a direct action on the heart, such as epinephrine, isoproterenol, dobutamine, calcium, glucagon, and digoxin.[80,81] α- and β-adrenergic receptors are not only intact, but the β-adrenergic receptor has been noted to become more sensitive to isoproterenol, perhaps due to β receptor up-regulation.[82] The response of the denervated heart to beta blockade has been shown to be similar to that of the innervated heart.[83]

The denervated heart does not respond to drugs that act indirectly, such as those mediated by the parasympathetic nervous system to decrease or increase vagal (cholinergic) tone. For example, atropine and pancuronium will have no effect on heart rate or AV node conduction, nor will anticholinesterases, such as edrophonium and neostigmine, reduce the heart rate and AV conduction. Carotid massage, phenylephrine, an ice bag on the face, and other efforts to stimulate the vagus nerve to decrease heart rate or convert a supraventricular tachycardia will have no effect.[84]

Drugs that act through direct and indirect mechanisms will produce only their direct effects. For example, the hypotensive effect of hydralazine, or any other direct-acting arterial dilator, will be amplified because there will be no reflex tachycardia. Digoxin has a positive inotropic effect but no acute effect on donor sinus rate or AV nodal conduction.[85] Long-term digoxin does decrease donor heart rate and AV conduction by direct effects. Despite its direct positive chronotropic and inotropic effects, the predominant vasoconstrictive effect of norepinephrine, which causes a marked increase in blood pressure, provokes reflex slowing of the heart rate in the innervated heart but not in the denervated heart.

Global Ischemia

Although denervation is permanent, the transplanted heart can recover from the global ischemia that occurs despite cold cardioplegic arrest at the time of procurement, the shortest possible ischemic time, and a sustained period of warm reperfusion prior to the discontinuation of bypass.[86] The result is a decrease in the diastolic compliance of both ventricles and a decrease in contractility, both in proportion to the degree of ischemia.[87] In the extreme case, the stroke volume becomes relatively fixed and the cardiac output becomes dependent upon the heart rate.[88]

It is important to understand the concept of diastolic compliance.[89] Any reduction in ventricular compliance changes the relationship between the ventricle's end-diastolic volume and the end-diastolic pressure, so that any given ventricular end-diastolic volume will have a higher end-diastolic pressure, and any given increase in end-diastolic volume will have a larger increase in end-diastolic pressure. Therefore, when assessing myocardial function by the Frank-Starling relationship, it must be recognized that if preload is measured by end-diastolic pressure (LVEDP, PAOP, PCWP, RVEDP, or CVP), rather than by end-diastolic volume, actual decreases in compliance will be interpreted as perceived decreases in contractility.

The newly transplanted heart will need high filling pressures to maintain an adequate preload during the immediate post-cardiopulmonary bypass period and perhaps for days until it has recovered and exhibits normal compliance.[12,90] Initially, right atrial pressures of 10–16 mmHg and left atrial pressures of 12–18 mmHg are required to optimize preload. Then, an acceptable cardiac output can usually be achieved with a constant infusion of isoproterenol to raise the heart rate from a slow sinus or nodal rhythm to a high-normal range based on the patient's age with its inotropic effect increasing the state of contractility. An optimal preload will prevent the need for excessive inotropic support and protect the patient from systemic hypotension occurring without a compensatory increase in heart rate when vasodilators are used to reduce afterload.

Susceptibility of the Right Ventricle to Increased Afterload

It is crucial to recognize the susceptibility of the right ventricle to the effects of the afterload imposed on it by the pulmonary vasculature.[24,26] The donor's normal right ventricle is a thin-walled, highly compliant, but poorly contractile structure with relatively little reserve to increase the force of contraction. Unlike the left ventricle, which maintains its stroke volume over a wide range of afterload, the stroke volume of the right ventricle decreases precipitously with small increments of afterload.[91] The reduced right ventricular ejection reduces the left ventricular preload, which reduces the cardiac output and the pulmonary blood flow. This, in turn, results in hypoxemia, hypercarbia, and lactic acidosis, in a vicious cycle that further increases the PA pressure and PVR.

It is this vulnerability that accounts for most of the intraoperative and early postoperative deaths, when the transplanted right ventricle acutely distends and fails as it is exposed for the first time to the increased PVR in the recipient.[37,42,92] Direct visualization will reveal a distended right ventricle with negligible wrinkling as it contracts. The PA, right ventricular, and central venous pressures will be high when, because of decreased delivery of blood to the lungs and the left side of the heart, the lungs may be pale and the pulmonary wedge, left atrial, and systemic blood pressures are low. In some cases, when the PA pressure, right ventricular end-diastolic volume, and right ventricular end-diastolic pressure are increased, the intraventricular septum may shift into the left ventricular cavity causing an "internal tamponade" with an elevated left ventricular end-diastolic pressure and further reduction in cardiac output.[93,94] The surgeon's preference for slightly oversized donor hearts for recipients with elevated pretransplant PVR is designed to reduce the risk of postoperative right heart failure.

Weaning from Cardiopulmonary Bypass

The conditions prior to weaning from cardiopulmonary bypass must be optimized so that the right ventricle is not allowed to distend (Table 4). The goal is to optimize therapy so bypass can be terminated with the first attempt, rather than to leisurely advance therapy as the right ventricle distends with each attempt to come off. It is fundamental to assure uniform rewarming to 34–36°C, a hematocrit around 28%–30%, profound anesthesia by administering morphine (1 mg/kg) into the pump to avoid light anesthesia and promote systemic and pulmonary vasodilatation, profound paralysis, 100% oxygen, alkalemia with the pH between 7.45 and 7.55, respiratory alkalosis with the PCO_2 between 25 and 30 mmHg,[26,28,95] and a normal sinus rhythm.

In every case, isoproterenol is begun in a dose of 0.1 μg/kg/min and increased usually to no higher than 5.0 μg/kg/min to obtain a heart rate that is top-normal for age (Fig. 1), which is an effective way to increase the cardiac output when the stroke volume is relatively fixed.[12,41,42,96] Isoproterenol will increase the state of contractility and help dilate the pulmonary vasculature; it may also help to convert the

Table 4 Weaning from Cardiopulmonary Bypass: Initial Pulmonary Vasodilator Therapy

Isoproterenol	0.1–5 μg/kg/min
Nitroprusside	1–5 μg/kg/min
Phentolamine	2–5 mg bolus
100% oxygen	
pH 7.45–7.55, PCO_2 25–30 mm Hg	
Profound anesthesia (morphine-1.0 mg/kg bolus)	
Profound paralysis	
Additional Pulmonary Vasodilator Therapy	
Amrinone	0.75 mg/kg bolus 5–10 μg/kg/min
Prostaglandin E_1 (via central venous catheter)	30–150 ng/kg/min
Preservation of Systemic Perfusion Pressure	
Norepinephrine	0.1–1 μg/kg/min
or	
Epinephrine	0.1–1 μg/kg/min
(via left atrial catheter)	

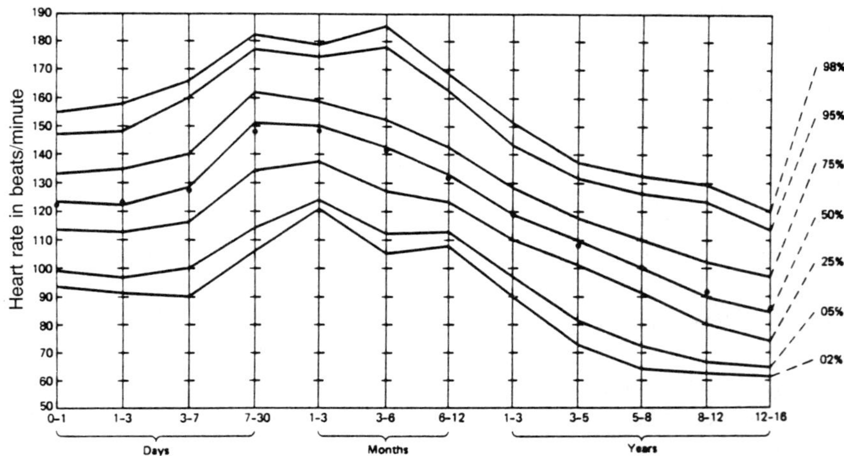

Figure 1: *Resting heart rates in normal children. Reproduced with permission from Davignon A, Rautaharju P, Boisselle E, et al: Normal ECG standards for infants and children. Pediatr Cardiol 1979/80, 1:123.*

most common dysrhythmia: a nodal rhythm that is sometimes difficult to diagnose with the recipient's P waves scattered throughout the ECG.[97] The diagnosis is usually made by looking directly at the heart for the sequence of contractions or by looking for cannon waves on the CVP tracing when the heart begins to eject. Isoproterenol is maintained to augment the cardiac output even when atrial or AV sequential pacing is necessary.[98] To facilitate rewarming and to enhance the cardiac output regardless of the preexisting vascular resistances, phentolamine is given in a bolus of 2–5 mg into the pump when rewarming is initiated and 1–5 μg/kg/min of nitroprusside is maintained in every patient.[37,99]

Frequently, additional inotropic support is required.[42,100] Because decreased left ventricular output decreases pulmonary blood flow and increases both PVR and the PA pressure–systemic arterial pressure ratio, an improvement in left ventricular performance will increase pulmonary blood flow and decrease PVR and the PA pressure–systemic arterial pressure ratio. Dopamine in doses of 5–10 μg/kg/min does not cause pulmonary vasoconstriction.[101] Rather, its beneficial effect on ventricular performance decreases the PVR and the PA pressure–systemic arterial pressure ratio, particularly when combined with a systemic vasodilator.[102] Dobutamine in doses of 5–10 μg/kg/min has a similar inotropic effect without causing vasoconstriction.[103–105]

As weaning from bypass is initiated and the preload is carefully optimized with right atrial pressures no higher than 10–16 mmHg and left atrial pressures no higher than 12–18 mmHg, particular attention is devoted to right ventricular function. Right ventricular failure resulting from excessive right ventricular afterload is suggested by minimal wrinkling of the right ventricle as it contracts and by excessive PA, right ventricular, and central venous pressures when there is a decrease in PA occluded pressures, left atrial pressures, and systemic blood pressures.

Pharmacologic pulmonary vasodilator therapy can then be increased aggressively to achieve maximal pulmonary vasodilatation (Table 4) so that the mean PA pressure is never allowed over about one-third of the mean systemic pressure and never above a mean of 25 mmHg. Amrinone may be added as a pulmonary vasodilator and as an inotrope in a bolus of 0.75 mg/kg over 2–3 min followed by 5–10 μg/kg/min.[106]

Prostaglandin E_1 is recognized as the most effective available pulmonary vasodilator, having been shown to lower the PVR and the PA pressure when other pulmonary vasodilators have failed.[12,107–109] Prostaglandin E_1 is administered by constant infusion through the CVP catheter or the PA catheter in a dose of 30–150 ng/kg/min (0.03–0.15 μg/kg/min). This dose range is about one-third of that normally used for maintaining ductal patency (0.1–4.0 μg/kg/min).[110]

These vasodilators, especially PGE_1, may cause profound systemic vasodilatation and systemic hypotension that may be offset by the infusion of norepinephrine or epinephrine, each in a dose of 0.1–1.0 μg/kg/min into the left atrium.[108] The rationale for this technique is that PGE_1 is almost completely metabolized by the lung when infused through the CVP or PA catheter. By administering a potent α-adrenergic agonist, with or without potent beta effects, through the left atrial catheter, the systemic vasodilatation with PGE_1 will be counteracted and the systemic perfusion pressure will be preserved. A left-sided infusion site avoids a bolus effect on the pulmonary vasculature and utilizes the metabolic capacity of the systemic capillary bed to remove some of the drug before it reaches the lung. It appears that PGE_1 released into the systemic circulation protects against the untoward renal and peripheral vascular effects of large doses of norepinephrine.

Failure to wean a patient from bypass requires a 15–30-min period of complete cardiopulmonary bypass without the use of inotropic agents to allow the donor heart to rest and recover while vasodilator therapy is optimized. It is also important to measure the transpulmonary valve gradient, the difference between the right ventricular systolic pressure and the PA systolic pressure, to rule out stenosis at the PA anastomosis as a cause of heart failure. When inotropic and vasodilator therapy fails,[111] mechanical support of the circulation by means of intrapulmonary, arterial balloon counterpulsation,[112] intra-aortic balloon counterpulsation,[113] or prolonged cardiopulmonary bypass is not likely to permit weaning of the transplanted heart before infection, renal failure, and/or pulmonary hypertension significantly reduce survival.[114]

Novitsky et al. reported an improved cardiac output and the need for less inotropic support in cardiac transplant recipients who had received T_3.[115] Observing that T_3 fell by a mean of 81% during the first 15 min after the initiation of cardiopulmonary bypass and remained low throughout the procedure, they assumed that acute depletion of T_3 might lead to metabolic changes similar to those seen in the brain-dead donor (abnormal mitochondrial function resulting in anaerobic metabolism and myocardial dysfunction).[5] They initially administered T_3 to 10 patients who had extremely poor myocardial function following bypass, and in each case, inotropic support was significantly reduced or discontinued. They subsequently began administering T_3 at the time of the release of the aortic cross clamp and reperfusion of the transplanted heart and noted excellent function in all 22 recipients. Our institution has not yet used T_3 for this purpose, awaiting controlled trials.

Regardless of how well the heart appears to perform, isoproterenol should not be completely discontinued for 2 or 3 days, because any period of bradycardia may lead to right and left ventricular distension from which it will be difficult to recover.[41] For example, if the patient is lightly anesthetized, but hyperdynamic, at the end of the procedure, the heart rate that is increased by circulating catecholamines will fall with the withdrawal of noxious stimulation.

It is also important to maintain pulmonary vasodilator therapy for a sustained period of time, perhaps 24 hours after the PA pressures are under control, because the labile pulmonary circulation is still capable of intense vasoconstriction. The criteria for extubation are the same as those applied to other open heart surgical patients, with most children who do well being extubated within 12–24 hours postoperatively. Although secondary pulmonary hypertension in a recipient resolves rapidly,[116] hypoxemia, hypercarbia, acidemia, excessive airway pressures, sympathetic stimulation, hypothermia, and hypervolemia must be avoided. Severe pulmonary hypertension should be treated with pharmacologic vasodilitation, controlled hyperventilation with 100% FiO_2 maintaining a PCO_2 of 25–30 mmHg, complete paralysis and anesthesia (pancuronium 0.1 mg/kg/hr and fentanyl 20 μg/kg/hr), and pulmonary toilet and stimulation.

References

1. Griepp RB, Stinson EB, Clark DA, et al:The cardiac donor. Surg Gynecol Obstet 1971, 133:795.
2. Guyton AC, Hall JE: Vasopressin and cardiovascular regulation. In Guyton AC, Hall JE, eds: Cardiovascular Physiology. University Park Press, Baltimore, 1982.
3. Richardson DW, Robinson AG: Desmopressin. Ann Intern Med 1985, 103:228.
4. Slapak M: The immediate care of potential donors for cadaveric organ transplantation. Anaesthesia 1978, 33:700.
5. Novitsky D, Cooper DK: Results of hormonal therapy in human brain-dead potential organ donors. Transplant Proc 1988, 20:59.
6. Levinson MM, Copeland JG: The organ donor: Physiology, maintenance, and procurement considerations. In Brown BR, ed: Anesthesia and Transplantation Surgery. Davis, Philadelphia, 1987:31.
7. Raferty AT, Johnson RW: Dopamine pretreatment in unstable kidney donors. Br Med J 1979, 1(6162):522.
8. Wetzel RC, Setzer N, Stiff JL, et al: Hemodynamic responses in brain-dead organ donor patients. Anesth Analg 1985, 64:125.
9. Copeland JG: Heart transplantation. In Cohn LH, ed: Modern Techniques in Surgery. Futura Publishing Co., Mount Kisco, NY, 1984, p. 1.
10. Colberg JE: En bloc excision of cadaver kidneys for transplantation. Arch Surg 1980, 115:1238.
11. Miller CH, Alexander JW, Smith EJ, et al: Salutary effect of phentolamine (Regitine) on renal vasoconstriction in donor kidneys: experimental and clinical studies. Transplantation 1974, 14:201.
12. Clark NJ, Martin RD: Anesthetic considerations for patients undergoing cardiac transplantation. J Cardiothorac Anesth 1988, 2:519.
13. Covell JW, Ross J: Nature and significance of alterations in myocardial compliance. Am J Cardiol 1973, 32:449.
14. Parmley WW: Pathophysiology of congestive heart failure. Am J Cardiol 1985, 56:7A.

15. Krueger JW: Fundamental mechanisms that govern cardiac function: A short review of cardiac sarcomere mechanics. Heart Failure 1988, 4: 137.
16. Francis G: Neurohumoral mechanisms involved in congestive heart failure. Am J Cardiol 1985, 55:15A.
17. Heinsimer JA, Lefkowitz RJ: The beta-adrenergic receptor in heart failure. Hosp Practice 1983, 73:103.
18. Bristow MR, Kantrowitz NE, Ginsburg R, et al: β-adrenergic function in heart muscle disease and heart failure. J Mol Cell Cardiol 1985, 17:41.
19. Fowler MB, Laser JA, Hopkins GL, et al: Assessment of the beta-adrenergic receptor pathway in the intact failing human heart: Progressive receptor down-regulation and subsensitivity to agonist response. Circulation 1986, 74:1290.
20. Ruffolo JR, Kopia GA: Importance of receptor regulation in the pathophysiology and therapy of congestive heart failure. Am J Med 1986, 80:67.
21. Bristow MR, Ginsburg R, Umans V, et al: β-1 and β-2 adrenergic receptor subpopulations in nonfailing and failing human ventricular myocardium: Coupling of both receptor subtypes to muscle contraction and selective β-1 receptor down- regulation in heart failure. Circ Res 1986, 59:297.
22. Ross J: Afterload mismatch and preload reserve: A conceptual framework for the analysis of ventricular function. Prog Cardiovasc Dis 1976, 18:255.
23. Weber KT, Janicki JS, Campbell C, et al: Pathophysiology of acute and chronic cardiac failure. Am J Cardiol 1987, 60:3C.
24. Weber KT, Janicki JS, Shroff SG, et al: The right ventricle: Physiologic and pathophysiologic considerations. Crit Care Med 1983, 11:323.
25. Malik AB, Kidd BS: Independent effects of changes in H+ and CO_2 concentrations on hypoxic pulmonary vasoconstriction. J Appl Physiol 1973, 34:318.
26. Burrows FA, Klinck JR, Rabinovitch M, et al: Pulmonary hypertension in children: Perioperative management. Can Anaesth Soc J 1986, 33:606.
27. Jenkins J, Lynn A, Edmonds J, et al: Effects of mechanical ventilation on cardiopulmonary function in children after open-heart surgery. Crit Care Med 1985, 13:77.
28. Drummond WH, Gregory GA, Heymann MA, et al: The independent effects of hyperventilation, tolazoline, and dopamine on infants with persistent pulmonary hypertension. J Pediatr 1981, 98:603.
29. Hickey PR: Anesthesia for neonatal orthotopic cardiac xenograft (editorial comment). J Cardiothorac Anesth 1987, 1:135.
30. Fowler MB, Schroeder JS: Current status of cardiac transplantation. Modern concepts of cardiovascular disease. 1986, 55:37.
31. Kormos RL, Thompson M, Hardesty MD, et al: Utility of preoperative right heart catheterization data as a predictor of survival after heart transplantation. (abstract) J Heart Trans 1986, 5:391.
32. Addonizio LJ, Gersony WM, Robbins RC, et al: Elevated pulmonary

vascular resistance and cardiac transplantation. Circulation 1987, 76(Suppl V):52.
33. Caves PK, Stinson EB, Billingham ME: Percutaneous transvenous endomyocardial biopsy in human heart recipients. Ann Thorac Surg 1973, 16:325.
34. Romano A, Niguidula FN: Technique of intraoperative placement of thermodilution catheter for cardiac output measurement in children. J Cardiovasc Surg 1980, 21:267.
35. Borland L: Allometric determination of the distance from the central venous pressure port to wedge position of balloon-tip catheters in pediatric patients. Crit Care Med 1986, 14:974.
36. Kay HR, Afshari M, Barash P, et al: Measurement of ejection fraction by thermal dilution techniques. J Surg Res 1983, 34:337.
37. Curling PE, Zaidan JR, Murphy DA, et al: Treatment of pulmonary hypertension after human orthotopic heart transplantation. Anesth Analg 1987, 66:537.
38. Michel L, Marsh HM, McMichan JC, et al: Infection of pulmonary artery catheters in critically ill patients. JAMA 1981, 245:1032.
39. Johnston WE, Prough DS, Royster RL, et al: Short-term sterility of the pulmonary artery catheter inserted through an external plastic shield. Anesth 1984, 61:461.
40. Garman JK: Anesthesia for cardiac transplantation. Cleveland Clinic Quart 1981, 48:142.
41. Ream AK, Fowles RE, Jamieson S. Cardiac transplantation. In Kaplan JA, ed: Cardiac Anesthesia. Grune & Stratton, Philadelphia, 1987, p. 881.
42. Hensley FA, Martin DE, Larach DR, et al: Anesthetic management for cardiac transplantation in North America—1986 survey. J Cardiothorac Anesth 1987, 1:429.
43. Hickey PR, Hansen DD: Fentanyl—and Sufentanil—oxygen-pancuronium anesthesia for cardiac surgery in infants. Anesth Analg 1984, 63: 117.
44. Hickey, PR, Hansen DD, Wessel DL, et al: Blunting of stress responses in the pulmonary circulation of infants by fentanyl. Anesth Analg 1985, 64:1137.
45. Davis PJ, Cook DR, Stiller RL, et al: Pharmacodynamics and pharmacokinetics of high-dose sufentanil in infants and children undergoing cardiac surgery. Anesth Analg 1987, 66:203.
46. Moore RA, Yang SS, McNicholas KW: Hemodynamic and anesthetic effects of sufentanil as the sole anesthetic for pediatric cardiac surgery. Anesth 1985, 62:725.
47. Hansen DD, Hickey PR: Anesthesia for hypoplastic left heart syndrome: Use of high-dose fentanyl in 30 neonates. Anesth Analg 1986, 65:127.
48. Stanley TH, Webster LR: Anesthetic requirements and cardiovascular effects of fentanyl-oxygen and fentanyl-diazepam-oxygen anesthesia in man. Anesth Analg 1978, 57:411.
49. Wynands JE, Wong P, Whalley DG, et al: Oxygen-fentanyl anesthesia in

patients with poor left ventricular function: Hemodynamics and plasma fentanyl concentrations. Anesth Analg 1983, 62:476.
50. Gallo JA, Cork RC: Anesthesia for cardiac transplantation. In Brown BR, ed: Anesthesia and Transplantation Surgery. Davis, Philadelphia, 1987, p. 91.
51. Demas K, Wyner J, Mihm FG, et al: Anaesthesia for heart transplantation: A retrospective study and review. Br J Anaesth 1986, 58:1357.
52. Massaut J, D'Hollander A, Barvais L, et al: Haemodynamic effects of midazolam in anaesthetized patients with coronary artery disease. Acta Anaesth Scand 1983, 27:299.
53. Reves J, Samuelson P, Lewis S: Midazolam maleate induction in patients with ischaemic heart disease: Haemodynamic observation. Can Anaesth Soc J 1979, 26:402.
54. Reves JG: Con: Benzodiazepines are not contraindicated as induction agents for coronary artery surgery. J Cardiothorac Anesth 1988, 2:844.
55. Tomicheck RC, Rosow CE, Philbin DM, et al: Diazepam-fentanyl interaction: Hemodynamic and hormonal effects in coronary artery surgery. Anesth Analg 1983, 62:881.
56. Howie MB: Pro: Benzodiazepines are contraindicated as induction agents for coronary artery surgery. J Cardiothor Anesth 1988, 2:841.
57. Ozinsky J: Cardiac transplantation—The anaesthetist's view: A case report. S Afr Med J 1967, 41:1268.
58. Reitz BA, Fowles RE, Ream AK: Cardiac transplantation. In Ream AK, Fogdall RP, eds: Acute Cardiovascular Management. Lippincott, Philadelphia, 1982:549.
59. Smith G: The effects of ketamine of the canine coronary circulation. Anaesth 1979, 34:555.
60. White PF, Way WL, Trevor AJ: Ketamine—Its pharmacology and therapeutic uses. Anesth 1982, 56:119.
61. Gooding JM, Dimick AR, Tavakoli M, et al: A physiologic analysis of cardiopulmonary response to ketamine anesthesia in non-cardiac patients. Anesth Analg 1977, 56:813.
62. Spotoft H, Horshin JD, Sorensen MB, et al: The cardiovascular effects of ketamine used for induction of anaesthesia in patients with valvular heart disease. Can Anaesth Soc J 1979, 26:463.
63. Mooray JP, Lynn AM, Stamm SJ, et al: Hemodynamic effects of ketamine in children with congenital heart diseases. Anesth Analg 1984, 63:895.
64. Hickey PR, Hansen DD, Cramolini GM, et al: Pulmonary and systemic hemodynamic responses to ketamine in infants with normal and elevated pulmonary vascular resistance. Anesth 1985, 62:287.
65. Waterman PM, Bjerke R: Rapid-sequence technique in patients with severe ventricular dysfunction. J Cardiothor Anesth 1988, 2:602.
66. Murkin JM, Moldenauer CC, Hug CC: High-dose fentanyl for rapid induction of anesthesia in patients with coronary artery disease. Can Anaesth Soc J 1985, 32:320.
67. Bazaral MG, Wagner R, Abi-Nader E, et al: Comparison of the effects of

15 and 60 μg/kg fentanyl used for induction of anesthesia in patients with coronary artery disease. Anesth Analg 1985, 64:312.
68. Zahl K, Ellison N: Influence of β-blockers on vecuronium/sufentanil or pancuronium/sufentanil combinations for rapid induction and intubation of cardiac surgical patients. J Cardiothor Anesth 1988, 2:607.
69. Lappas DG, Buckley MJ, Laver MB, et al: Left ventricular performance and pulmonary circulation following addition of nitrous oxide to morphine during coronary artery surgery. Anesth 1975, 43:61.
70. Lunn JK, Stanley TH, Eisele J, et al: High dose fentanyl anesthesia for coronary artery surgery: Plasma fentanyl concentrations and influence of nitrous oxide on cardiovascular responses. Anesth Analg 1979, 58: 390.
71. Eisele JH, Reitan JA, Massumi RA: Myocardial performance and N_2O analgesia in coronary artery diseases. Anesth 1976, 44:16.
72. Schulte-Sasse U, Hess W, Tarnow J: Pulmonary vascular responses to nitrous oxide in patients with normal and high pulmonary vascular resistance. Anesth 1982, 57:9.
73. Hilgenberg JC, McCammon RL, Stoelting RK: Pulmonary and systemic vascular resistance responses to nitrous oxide in patients with mitral stenosis and pulmonary hypertension. Anesth Analg 1980, 59:323.
74. Hickey PR, Hansen DD, Strafford M, et al: Pulmonary and systemic hemodynamic effects of nitrous oxide in infants with normal and elevated pulmonary vascular resistance. Anesth 1986, 65:374.
75. Shaver JA, Leon DF, Gray S, et al: Hemodynamic observations after cardiac transplantation. N Engl J Med 1969, 281:822.
76. Goodman DJ, Rossen RM, Rider AK, et al: The effect of cycle length on cardiac refractory periods in the denervated human heart. Am Heart J 1976, 91:332.
77. Bexton RS, Nathan AW, Hellestrand KJ, et al: The electrophysiologic characteristics of the transplanted human heart. Am Heart J 1984, 107:1.
78. Kent KM, Cooper TC: The denervated heart. A model for studying autonomic control of the heart. N Engl J Med 1974, 291:1017.
79. Pope SE, Stinson EB, Daughters GT, et al: Exercise response of the denervated heart in long-term cardiac transplant recipients. Am J Cardiol 1980, 46:213.
80. Fowles RE, Reitz BA, Ream AK: Drug actions in a transplanted or artificial heart. In Kaplan JA, ed: Cardiac Anesthesia. Vol II: Cardiovascular Pharmacology. Grune & Stratton, Orlando, 1983, p. 641.
81. Kavanagh T, Yacoub MH, Mertens DJ, et al: Cardiorespiratory responses to exercise training after orthotopic cardiac transplantation. Circulation 1988, 77:162.
82. Lurie KG, Bristow MR, Reitz BA: Increased β-adrenergic receptor density in an experimental model of cardiac transplantation. J Thorac Cardiovasc Surg 1983, 86:195.
83. Cannom DS, Rider AK, Stinson EB, et al: Electrophysiological studies in the denervated transplanted human heart. II. Response to norepinephrine, isoproterenol and propranolol. Am J Cardiol 1975, 36:859.

84. Cannom DS, Graham AF, Harrison DC: Electrophysiological studies in the denervated transplanted human heart. Circ Res 1973, 32:268.
85. Ricci DR, Orlick AE, Reitz BA, et al: Depressant effect of digoxin on atrioventricular conduction in man. Circulation 1978, 57:898.
86. Greenberg ML, Uretsky BF, Reddy PS, et al: Long-term hemodynamic follow-up of cardiac transplant patients treated with cyclosporine and prednisone. Circulation 1985, 71:487.
87. Novitsky D, Cooper D, Boniaszcuk J, et al: The significance of left ventricular volume measurement after heart transplantation using radionuclide techniques. Heart Trans 1985, 4:206.
88. Young JB, Leon CA, Short HD, et al: Evolution of hemodynamics after orthotopic heart and heart-lung transplantation: Early restrictive patterns persisting in occult fashion. J Heart Trans 1987, 6:34.
89. Sibbald WJ, Calvin J, Driedger AA: Right and left ventricular preload and diastolic ventricular compliance: Implications for therapy in critically ill patients. In: Critical Care: State of the Art. Fullerton, CA, Society of Critical Care Medicine, 1982, vol 3:F1-F33.
90. Greenberg ML, Uretsky BF, Reddy PS, et al: Long-term hemodynamic follow-up of cardiac transplant patients treated with cyclosporine and prednisone. Circulation 1985, 71:487.
91. McFadden ER, Braunwald E: Cor pulmonale. In Braunwald E, ed: Heart Disease and Assessment. WB Saunders, Philadelphia, 1984, pp. 1597–1616.
92. Reves JG: Anesthesia and cardiac transplantation. In Stanley TH, Petty WC, eds: Anesthesia and the Cardiovascular System. Martinus Nijhoff, Boston, 1984, p. 217.
93. Jardin F, Farcot JC, Boisanti C, et al: Influence of positive end-expiratory pressure on left ventricular performance. N Engl J Med 1981, 304: 387.
94. Prewitt RM, Ghignone M: Treatment of right ventricular dysfunction in acute respiratory failure. Crit Care Med 1983, II:346.
95. Peckham GJ, Fox WW: Physiologic factors affecting pulmonary artery pressure in infants with persistent pulmonary hypertension. J Pediatr 1978, 93:1005.
96. Nakatsuka M, Colquhoun AD, Barnhart G: Right ventricular function of the denervated heart immediately after heart transplantation. (abstract) In: Proceedings of the 1989 Annual Meeting of the Society of Cardiovascular Anesthesiologists. Seattle, 1989, p. 231.
97. Schroeder JS, Berke DK, Graham AF, et al: Arrhythmias after cardiac transplantation. Am J Cardiol 1974, 33:604.
98. Ingels NB, Ricci DR, Daughters GT, et al: Effects of heart rate augmentation on left ventricular volumes and cardiac output of the transplanted human heart. Circulation 1977, 56(Suppl II):32.
99. Wyner J, Finch EL: Heart and Heart-lung transplantation. In Gelman S, ed: Anesthesia and Organ Transplantation. WB Saunders, Philadelphia, 1987, p. 111.

100. Grebenik CR, Robinson PN: Cardiac transplantation at Harefield. A review from the anaesthetist's stand-point. Anaesthesia 1985, 40:131.
101. Williams DB, Kiernan PD, Schaff HV, et al: The hemodynamic response to dopamine and nitroprusside following right atrium-pulmonary artery bypass (Fontan procedure). Ann Thorac Surg 1982:34:51.
102. Hayman AL, Lippton HL, Ignarro LJ, et al: Analysis of autonomic response in the pulmonary vascular bed. In Said SI, ed: The Pulmonary Circulation and Acute Lung Injury. Futura Publishing Co., Mount Kisco, NY, 1985.
103. Perkin RM, Levin DL, Webb R, et al: Dobutamine: A hemodynamic evaluation in children in shock. J Pediatr 1982, 100:977.
104. Bohn DJ, Poirier CS, Edmonds JF, et al: Hemodynamic effects of dobutamine after cardiopulmonary bypass in children. Crit Care Med 1980, 8:367.
105. Zaritsky A, Chernow B: Catecholamines in critical care medicine. Crit Care Q 1983, 6:39.
106. Colucci WS, Wright RF, Braunwald E: New positive inotropic agents in the treatment of congestive heart failure. N Engl J Med 1986, 314:290, 349.
107. Dewhirst WE: Prostaglandin E_1 for refractory right heart failure after coronary artery bypass grafting. J Cardiothor Anesth 1988, 2:56.
108. D'Ambra MN, LaRaia PJ, Philbin DM, et al: Prostaglandin E_1: A new therapy for refractory right heart failure and pulmonary hypertension after mitral valve replacement. J Thorac Cardiovasc Surg 1985, 89:567.
109. Armitage JM, Hardesty RL, Griffith BP: Prostaglandin E_1: An effective treatment of right heart failure after orthotopic heart transplantation. J Heart Transplant 1987, 6:348.
110. Silone ED: Administration of E-type prostaglandins in ductus-dependent congenital heart disease. Pediatr Cardiol 1982, 2:303.
111. Reves JG: Vasoactive drugs and when to use them. In Thomas SJ, ed: Manual of Cardiac Anesthesia. Churchill Livingstone, New York, 1984, p. 35.
112. Miller DC, Moreno-Cabral RT, Stinson EB, et al: Pulmonary artery balloon counterpulsation for acute right ventricular infarction. J Thorac Cardiovasc Surg 1980, 80:760.
113. Farrar D, Compton P, Hershon J, et al: Right ventricular function in an operating room model of mechanical left ventricular assistance and its effects in patients with depressed ventricular function. Circulation 1985, 72:1279.
114. Kanter KR, Pennington DG, McBride LR, et al: Mechanical circulatory assistance after heart transplantation. J Heart Trans 1987, 6:150.
115. Novitsky D, Cooper DK, Zuhdi N: Triiodothyronine therapy in the cardiac transplant recipient. Transplant Proc 1988, 20:65.
116. Bhatia SJ, Kirshenbaum JM, Shemin RJ, et al: Time course of resolution of pulmonary hypertension and right ventricular remodeling after orthotopic cardiac transplantation. Circulation 1987, 76(4):819.

Chapter 6

Operative Considerations

Jeffrey M. Dunn and Pierantonio Russo

Donor Procedure

Despite the great gains in the cardiac transplant arena, perhaps the most exasperating aspect remains the paucity of acceptable donors. Indeed, despite the increased population awareness, number of transplant programs, and potential recipients, the number of cardiac transplants performed has begun to tail off, increasing the discrepancy between the number of potential recipients and donors. Essential for a successful program is a well-organized procurement system. Criteria for, and declaration of, brain death is the responsibility of the hospital and physicians caring for the potential donor. The United Network for Organ Sharing has developed criteria for appropriate distribution by a uniform and equitable system taking into account the geographic location of the donor and recipient, the recipient condition and urgency for an organ, and length of time the potential recipient has been awaiting an organ. These criteria undergo continued adjustment and refinement. In addition, some latitude is present for use of an organ among transplant centers and potential recipients within a designated procurement area.

Frequently, the donor heart must be procured from a distant site. Transportation logistics and coordination with other transplant teams in the multiorgan procurement is best organized by the local organ procurement program—in our area, the Delaware Valley Organ Procurement Organization.

Donor Criteria

The criteria for an acceptable donor organ include the status of the donor heart as well as the appropriateness of the heart for the specific recipient in mind (Table 1). Needless to say, the competence of the donor heart is of prime concern. The donor heart should support adequate hemodynamic circulation in the donor without the reliance of inotropic agents other than in the early resuscitative period. Continued hypotension, acidosis or other signs of low cardiac output are of grave concern. Such events may indicate a poorly functioning heart. In addition, prolonged acidosis, hypotension, and hemodynamic shock may produce ischemic cardiac changes in an otherwise good donor organ, rendering it unsuitable for use. Other indications of a poor donor organ may include chest trauma, ECG changes, and arrhythmias. The echocardiogram is most useful in diagnosing pericardial effusions, akinetic cardiac muscle, myocardial failure, and even coincidental congenital cardiac defects. With a normal ECG and echocardiogram, accompanying normal hemodynamics, and the absence of a positive cardiovascular history, once can expect a good heart for transplantation. The heart must be further examined at the time of explantation for coronary artery disease and contusions. In rare cases, organ acceptability can be expanded beyond 40 to 45 years of age. When it becomes necessary to use an older heart in urgent situations, further evaluation may include cardiac catheterization. We have not found the need for such older donors in our pediatric transplantation experience.

It is not uncommon for the brain-dead donor to demonstrate periods of severe hypotension. During these episodes, inotropic agents may be necessary. These episodes are most often secondary to hypovolemia or peripheral vascular instability. When they occur, they can

Table 1 Donor Criteria

Age—less than 45 years
Size—20% range of recipient weight
Tumor-free (except CNS)
Infection-free*
No cardiac disease*
No cardiac trauma
Hemodynamically stable*

*These are individually evaluated so as not to categorically reject a donor.

be expected to respond to volume management, and inotropes can then be weaned.

Other criteria that may be contraindications to cardiac transplantation include infection or sepsis, malignancy (other than CNS), and other communicable disease such as hepatitis or HIV.

The specific appropriateness of matching a donor and recipient is of utmost importance. Major ABO comparability is essential because of preformed recipient antibodies. Rh compatibility is probably not essential, and we frequently transplant Rh(+) organs to Rh(−) recipients. The importance of matching HLA antigens is questionable. The HLA antigens are either polypeptides (HLA-A, -B, and -C) or glycoproteins (HLA-D and -DR). Although we perform HLA typing of both the donor and recipient, this is mainly for retrospective data analysis at our center, and we do not use this information to prospectively help match donor with recipient.

Most recipients do not carry preformed cytotoxic antibodies. These antibodies probably are secondary to previous antigen contact such as from blood transfusions. A "cytotoxic screen" against a random panel of cells is performed routinely on all potential recipients. If the percent reactivity is greater than 5% to 15%, a crossmatch against the potential donor is essential to avoid a hyperacute reaction. We do not carry out a donor–recipient crossmatch when the cytotoxic screen demonstrates no reactivity.

Finally, size match between the donor and recipient is essential. If the donor heart is too small, low cardiac output and cardiac failure can be expected. A too large heart may not successfully fit in a smaller mediastinum. In our adult and older children, a 20-kg discrepancy in either direction is probably acceptable. In a small infant or child, this formula is overly generous. In general, a heart from a donor 20% larger or smaller than the recipient will be easily accommodated in the recipient mediastinum and provide adequate cardiac output.

Donor Management

Medical management of the donor is essential after the declaration of brain death to maintain a healthy donor organ. Hypotension must be managed with appropriate fluid replacement and transient inotropic support. Acid–base and electrolyte balance are equally important. This may be a challenge in the donor with diabetes insipidus secondary to CNS damage. The high urine output of diabetes insipidus is managed with appropriate fluid and electrolyte replacement as well as vasopressin.

Organ Procurement Procedure

The procurement procedure requires the interdisciplinary coordination not only of operating room personnel and anesthesiologists one is not used to working with, but most often of other transplant surgeons removing other organs: kidneys, liver, pancreas, and even bowel. Coordination of the procedure is therefore of utmost importance. Preoperative cooperation is the rule, and in virtually all cases, modification of each team's protocol can be accomplished to everyone's satisfaction.

The donor is placed in the supine position. An arterial and central venous line are essential. The central line is positioned such that it can be removed just prior to removal of the heart. The sternum and abdomen are prepped and draped sterilely. A median sternotomy is performed, and extended into the abdomen if other organs are to be taken. The pericardium is opened anteriorly, and the heart is marsupialized in a pericardial cradle. The heart is gently explored externally for coronary artery plaques or calcification and for contusions. The heart is gently raised to examine the left ventricle posteriorly.

The ascending aorta and superior (SVC) and inferior vena cavae (IVC) are isolated on snares. A pursestring suture for cardioplegia is placed on the ascending aorta just below the innominate artery. In small hearts, the cardioplegia site can be the innominate artery itself to preserve maximum length of the ascending aorta. In pediatric donors, a patent ductus arteriosus may be suspected or confirmed by echocardiogram. If so, it can be isolated via the mediastinum and ligated just prior to cardioplegia delivery. If multiple organs are to be removed, the heart is gently covered with a damp gauze and the abdominal dissection can begin. The cardiac dissection is adequate to allow rapid cooling and removal of the heart from this point on if the donor becomes unstable.

Systemic cooling or systemic vasodilators are to be avoided prior to removal of the heart, although they may be part of a protocol for isolated removal of the kidneys or liver.

With completion of the dissection for the abdominal organs and placement of abdominal vessel cannulae, attention is again turned to the mediastinum. Sodium heparin (3 mg/kg) is given intravenously. The central venous line is withdrawn to above the superior vena cava to avoid its transection as the heart is excised. A cardioplegia needle (14F angiocath) is placed in the ascending aorta through the previously placed pursestring suture. The superior vena cava is ligated high in the mediastinum with a 2-0 Dacron ligature. The inferior vena cava is clamped close to the diaphragm. The decreased venous return results in a drop in systemic pressure, at which time the ascending aorta is crossclamped distal to the cardioplegia needle. Cardioplegia is begun slowly by pressurizing the cardioplegia bag. Simultaneously, the inferior vena cava is divided on the cardiac side of the IVC clamp, and a left pulmonary vein is divided (Fig. 1). These provide decompression of both the left and right ventricles. Warm blood is aspirated from the mediastinum, and the heart is bathed in an iced slush. Cardiac relaxation should ensue within a few seconds of beginning cardioplegia. A total of 30 cc/kg of cardioplegia is instilled. We utilize a crystalloid solution of 1,000 cc D5W, 80 mEq KCl, 12.5 gm mannitol, and 25 mEq $NcHCO_3$. When the abdominal organs are to be removed, the liver-kidney procurement team prefers to decompress the inferior vena cava to avoid organ congestion. This can be accomplished by aspiration cannulae in the abdominal vena cava or by partial decompression via the vena caval division in the mediastinum. When decompression is partially into the mediastinal route, care must be taken to discard this warm blood less it rewarm the heart.

With completion of the cardioplegia infusion in the aortic route, the heart is excised. The superior vena cava is divided above the previous ligature to avoid damage to the sinoatrial node. The remaining pulmonary veins are likewise sharply divided. The aorta is divided just proximal to the cross clamp. The left and right pulmonary arteries are divided just beyond the main pulmonary artery bifurcation. The excess aortic and pulmonary tissue can be easily trimmed during the implantation procedure. The extra length may be helpful for anastomosis in congenital heart disease with abnormal great vessel relations. The heart is ready to be removed. Some fibrous connections between the posterior left atrium and pericardial reflections are a constant finding and require sharp division. The heart can now be removed to the back table for preparation for transport.

The heart is bathed in cold (4°C) cardioplegia in a basin. The left atrium is examined. An incision is made between each of the pulmonary vein orifices to create a single left atriotomy (Fig. 2). The heart is

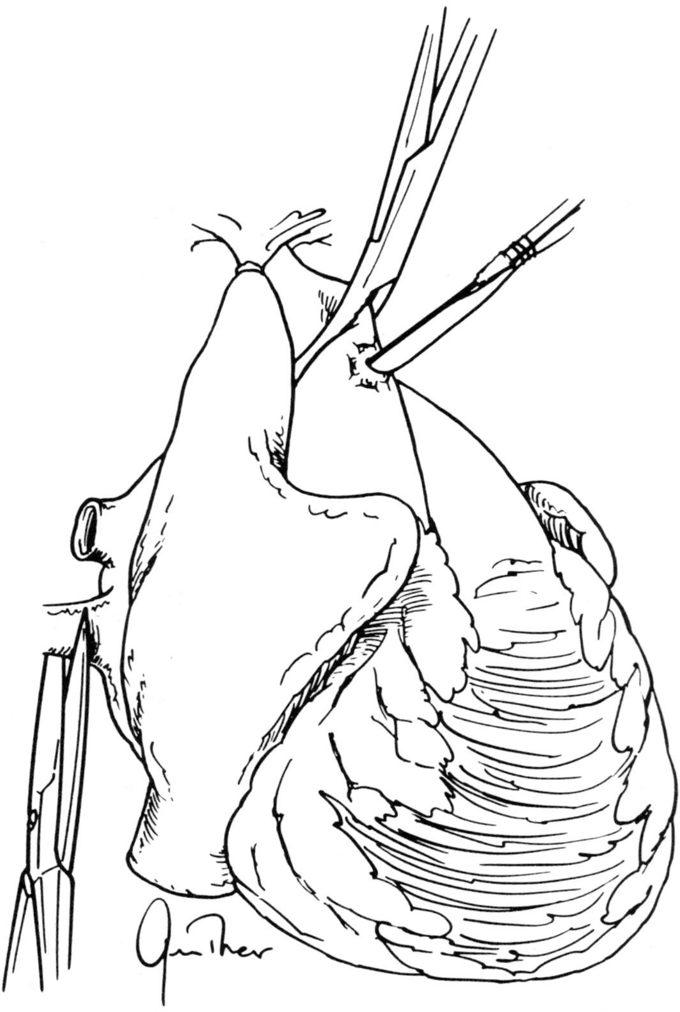

Figure 1: *Donor heart during excision. Cardioplegia is instilled by a 14-gauge catheter in the ascending aorta. An aortic cross clamp is distal to the cardioplegia catheter. The superior vena cava has been ligated, and the inferior vena cava is divided for decompression of the right heart. The illustration shows a pulmonary vein being divided for left heart decompression.*

placed with cold cardioplegia solution in a sterile plastic container that, in turn, is placed in three, consecutive, sterile bowel bags. This container is placed in a ice-filled Igloo Cooler for transport.

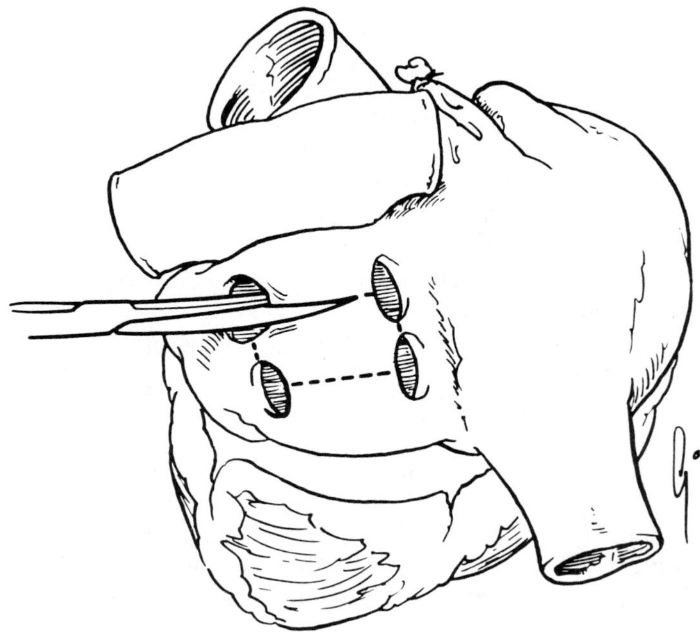

Figure 2: *The excised donor heart, posterior view. A window is incised between the four pulmonary venous os to create a single, large communication for anastomosis to the recipient left atrial cuff.*

Table 2 Procurement Pack

Instruments*	Cardioplegia Supplies
2 DeBakey forceps	5 vials 40 mEq KCl
1 Long Russion forceps	5 vials Mannitol 25%
1 Long right-angle clamp (Mixter)	3 amps $NaHCO_3$ (50 mEq)
2 Glover coarctation clamps	3 60-cc syringes
2 Schmidt toncel forceps	3 30-cc syringes
2 Crile hemostats	4 1,000-cc bags DSW
1 Metzenbaum scissors	Pressure infusion
1 Lebshe knife	3 3-W stopcocks
1 Orthopaedic mallet	14F angiocath
1 Favalora-Morse sternal retractor	5 bowel bags
	1 sterile jar
	1 Igloo Cooler with ice

*These instruments are used to compliment those of general surgical trays at the donor hospital.

Pediatric Considerations

In general, the donor procedure parallels the procedures in adult transplantation. The donor, like the recipient, will frequently be from the pediatric population. Persistent fetal and neonatal communications—patent ductus arteriosus and patent foramen ovale (PFO)—are more likely to be present in a pediatric donor. The donor evaluation, including physical examination and echocardiogram, should elicit these findings. When present, they are easily identified and corrected during the donor procurement.

A patent ductus should be isolated and ligated prior to infusion of cardioplegia. This is performed from the mediastinal approach during organ procurement.[1] With gentle inferior traction on the main pulmonary artery, blunt and sharp dissection is utilized to isolate the ductus on a #2 silk ligature. Once isolated, the donor procurement is carried out as reviewed above. After ligation of the superior vena cava and clamping the inferior vena cava, the ductus is ligated during the period of systemic hypotension just before the aorta is crossclamped and cardioplegia is introduced. Ductal ligation during this hypotension is more easily performed with a reduced risk of rupture of the friable ductal tissue.

The PFO may be hemodynamically insignificant in the donor, but may produce significant shunting after transplantation, especially in the noncompliant posttransplanted heart or during transient right heart failure. It is easily closed on the back table prior to implantation. The PFO is readily exposed through the left atriotomy produced by incising the atrium between the pulmonary veins. The PFO is identified and closed with a figure-of-eight or mattress suture of 4-0 Dacron or polypropylene. Alternately, the PFO can be exposed or visualized via the inferior vena caval opening, especially if this is enlarged prior to implantation. A larger PFO or a secundum or sinus venous atrial septal defect can likewise be closed primarily or with a small patch of pericardium or Gortex. These lesions should not be contraindications to organ donation unless they are associated with donor heart hypertrophy, dilatation, or cardiac failure, which occurs rarely.

To our knowledge, a donor heart with a ventricular septal defect has not been used clinically for transplantation. Again, this need not be a contraindication to transplantation. A small defect with minimal hemodynamic consequence and normal myocardial function should be an appropriate donor organ. The defect should be readily repairable through the tricuspid valve after explantation. More complex cardiac lesions, especially with secondary ventricular dysfunction, should be considered a contraindication to transplantation.

The donor procurement may also be altered because of the underlying cardiac status of the recipient. Hypoplastic left heart syndrome is the most obvious example of this and will be discussed separately in another chapter. Other congenital lesions that have been transplanted include single-ventricle status post-Fontan and transposed great vessels. In general, we attempt to remove the aortic arch, the main and branch pulmonary arteries, and generous portions of the superior and inferior vena cavae to allow for modifications of the implantation. The branch pulmonary arteries are especially useful in reconstruction of previously manipulated recipient pulmonary arteries and to enlarge the pulmonary artery anastomosis to prevent stricture with recipient growth (Fig. 3). Long segments of the donor aorta and pulmonary artery allow for aortic and pulmonary anastomosis in recipients with transposed or otherwise malrotated great vessels without the use of prosthetic material. Needless to say, the specific technique of implantation should be anticipated preoperatively in cases of com-

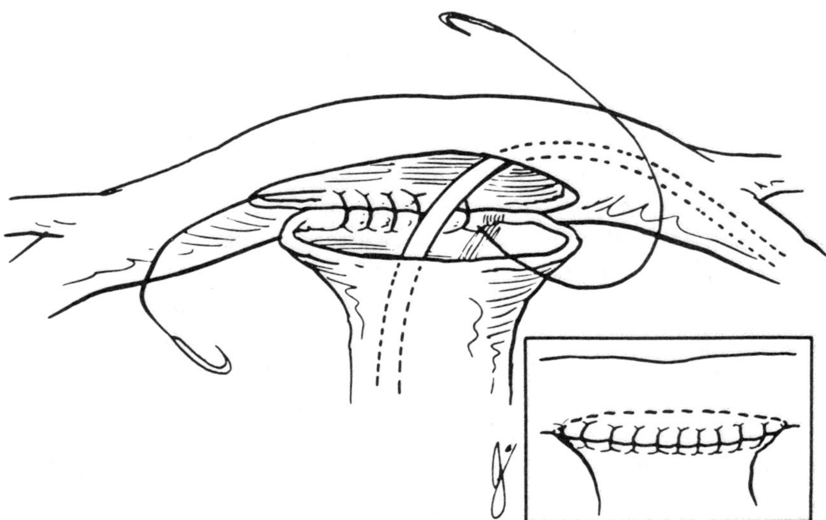

Figure 3: *Demonstrates the use of a splayed donor right and left pulmonary artery to enlarge the pulmonary anastomosis.*

plex congenital defects in the recipient, and the donor explantation modified appropriately.

Recipient Procedure

Operative Technique

Communication between the donor and recipient team is essential. By protocol, our donor team contacts the recipient team at the following intervals:

1. Upon arrival at the donor hospital and after initial evaluation of the donor. The quality of the heart and an estimated time of explantation and return to the recipient hospital is reported.
2. Upon surgical inspection of the donor heart after donor median sternotomy. Again, a revised estimate of explantation and arrival time is reported to the recipient surgical team.
3. After explantation and during back-table preparation of the heart. A final update on expected arrival time is reported.
4. During transit, about 1/2 hour before expected arrival at the recipient hospital.

In most cases, the procedures parallels that in the adult population.[2,3] The recipient procedure is started and coordinated, based on expected time of arrival of the donor heart and the anticipated time required for induction of anesthesia and institution of cardiopulmonary bypass. After induction of anesthesia, a pulmonary artery catheter is floated into the main pulmonary artery. It may be useful during the early phases of the procedure in the recipient with low cardiac output and will ultimately be repositioned during implantation of the donor heart. A median sternotomy is performed, and the heart marsupialized in a pericardial cradle. The ascending aorta and main pulmonary artery are dissected free from each other from the level of the aortic root to the innominate artery. Umbilical tape is placed around the ascending aorta, and snared tapes around the superior and inferior vena cava.

Cardiopulmonary bypass is instituted when the donor heart arrival is imminent (Fig. 4). Sodium heparin (3 mg/kg) is given intravenously, either through a central venous catheter by the anesthesiolo-

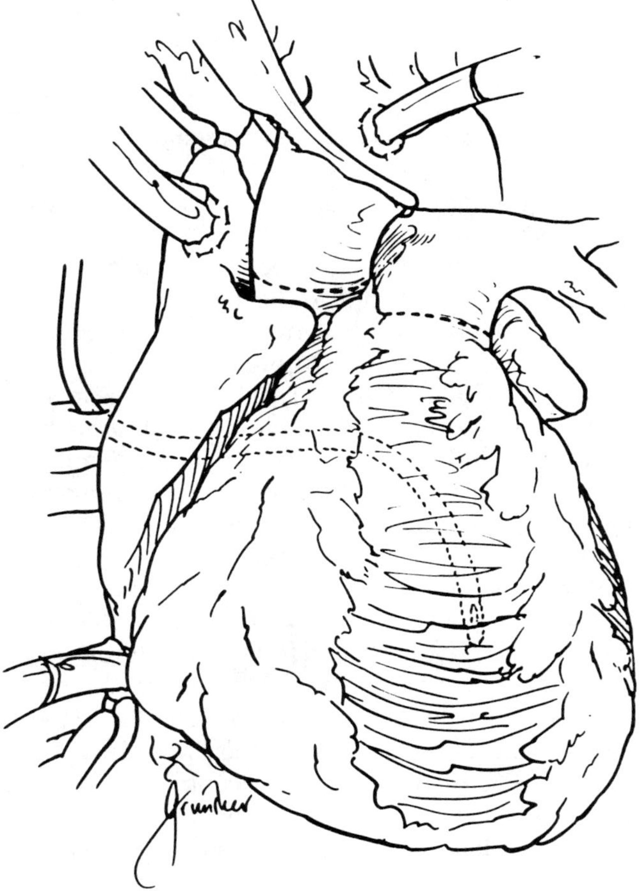

Figure 4: *Recipient heart on bypass, ready for excision. The aortic perfusion cannula is in the distal ascending or proximal arch of the aorta, adjacent to the innominate artery to provide an adequate aortic cuff below. The vena cavae are cannulated separately, through either the cavae themselves or the right atrium adjacent to the cavae. A left ventricular sump is shown entering the superior right pulmonary vein and coursing through the left atrium, across the mitral valve, and into the left ventricle.*

gist or via the right atrial appendage by the surgeon. The aorta, SVC, and IVC are cannulated through pursestrings. The aorta is cannulated high on the ascending aorta just below the innominate artery. The SVC and IVC are separately cannulated through pursestring sutures in the body of the right atrium close to the respective cavae. We have found right-angled catheters (Riggs or DLP) to be most convenient. Cardiopulmonary bypass is instituted with a crystalloid and blood prime predicted to produce a hematocrit of 20% on bypass. Cardiopulmonary bypass is maintained at a cardiac index of 2.2 L/min and the patient is moderately cooled to 26–28°C. A sump drain is placed through the superior right pulmonary vein into the left atrium or the left ventricle if there are no LV thrombi.

When the donor heart is available, the recipient heart can be excised. The aorta is crossclamped. The ascending aorta and pulmonary artery are just above the respective aortic and pulmonary valves. The atria are then divided starting at the right atrial appendage. The appendage is removed and the right atrial free wall is incised parallel and adjacent to the atrioventricular groove. The atrial septum and left atrial free wall are then incised in a like manner, removing the left atrial appendage. The recipient heart can then be removed (Fig. 5). Care is taken to excise and remove the coronary sinus adjacent to the left atrioventricular groove. If it is not completely removed, or if the os of the coronary sinus is left in place with the retained atrial cuffs, care must be taken to incorporate them in the atrial anastomosis.

The donor heart is then removed from its cold transport media and brought to the operative field. The left atrium is anastomosed first using a 28-inch, 4-0 polypropylene suture. The anastomosis begins joining the recipient left atrial cuff at the level of the superior left pulmonary vein to the donor atrium adjacent to the donor left atrial appendage (Fig. 6). The donor heart is delivered into the mediastinum adjacent to the recipient cuff, and the anastomosis is continued caudally, anastomosing the posterior or free wall of the left atrium. The other limb of the running suture is carried cephalad and onto the atrial septum. We prefer a double-layer anastomosis of the atrial septum, although others utilize a single layer. This is accomplished by incorporating the full thickness of the medial donor left atrium, but partial thickness of the recipient septum including the left atrial endothelium. Before completion of the left atrial anastomosis, the LV sump lying in the donor left atrium is advanced through the mitral valve into the donor left ventricle.

The right atrial anastomosis is performed next. The donor right atrial incision is enlarged from the orifice of the inferior vena cava up the body of the right atrium adjacent to the septal anastomosis and toward the donor right atrial appendage (Fig. 7). This incision is en-

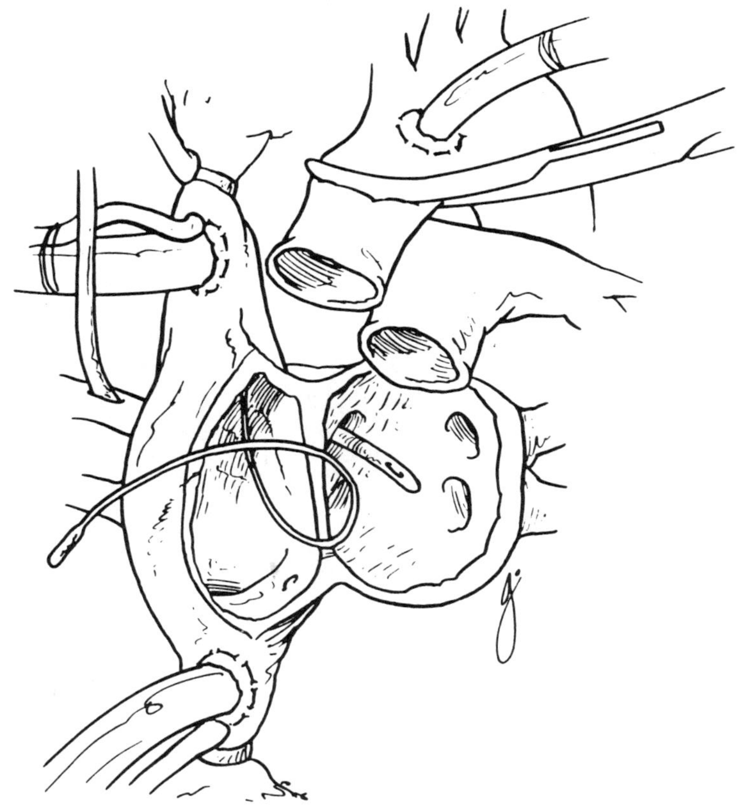

Figure 5: *Recipient mediastinum after excision of the recipient old heart. A large cuff of left and right atrium remains. The atrial appendages have been excised. Note the long length of ascending aorta and main pulmonary artery. This length is needed for orienting the aortic and pulmonary anastomosis in patients with malrotated great vessels. The Swan-Ganz pulmonary catheter is shown coursing from the superior vena cava and the LV vent is shown entering the left atrial remnant from the superior right pulmonary veins. These catheters will be replaced in the pulmonary artery and LV, respectively, during the implantation of the donor heart.*

larged to correspond to the size of the recipient right atrial cuff. The anastomosis begins at the inferior portion of the atrial septum, again incorporating full-thickness donor atrium with partial-thickness recipient septum. Before completion of the right atrial anastomosis, the Swan-Ganz catheter is advanced through the donor tricuspid valve, right ventricle, and pulmonary artery into the free mediastinum. It will

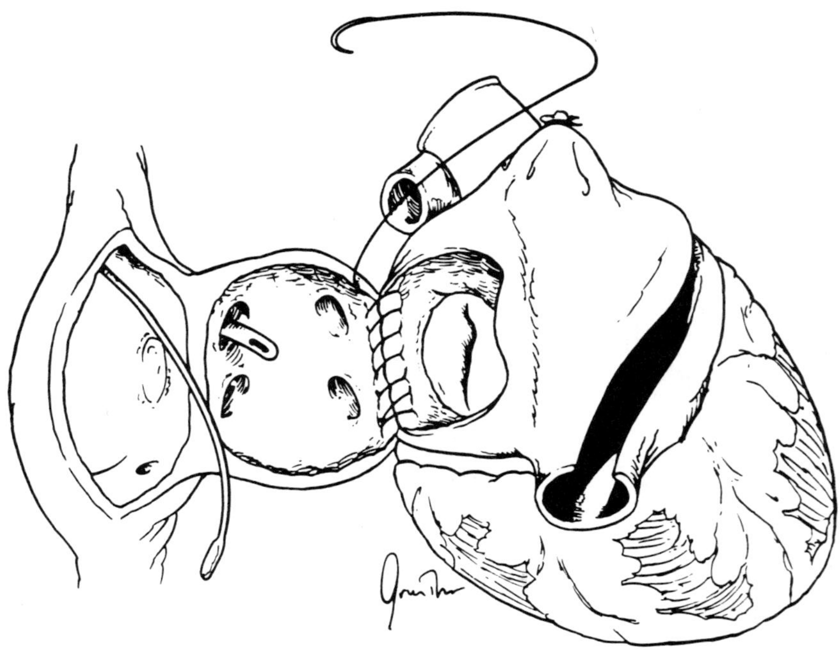

Figure 6: *Left atrial anastomosis. The implantation is begun with anastomosis of the donor left atrial window to the recipient left atrial cuff. The anastomosis begins adjacent to the donor left atrial appendage and recipient superior left pulmonary vein. Before completion of this anastomosis, the LV sump (shown here in the left atrium) is passed through the donor mitral valve into the left ventricle. An incision from the open donor inferior vena cava, up superiorly, parallel to the atrial septum, and toward the atrial appendage, is made to accept the large donor atrial cuff.*

be positioned in the distal recipient pulmonary artery later. The right atrial anastomosis is completed. If the recipient coronary sinus os remains, care must be taken to incorporate it into the right atrial chamber or anastomosis.

The pulmonary anastomosis is accomplished with a single-layer, simple, 4-0 polypropylene suture after positioning the Swan-Ganz catheter. This is facilitated by placing the posterior layer of the anastomosis first, placing the pulmonary catheter across the anastomosis, and then completing the anterior row. The aortic anastomosis is completed last. We utilize a two-layer closure. The first layer an averting mattress, the second, a simple running suture, both with 4-0 polypro-

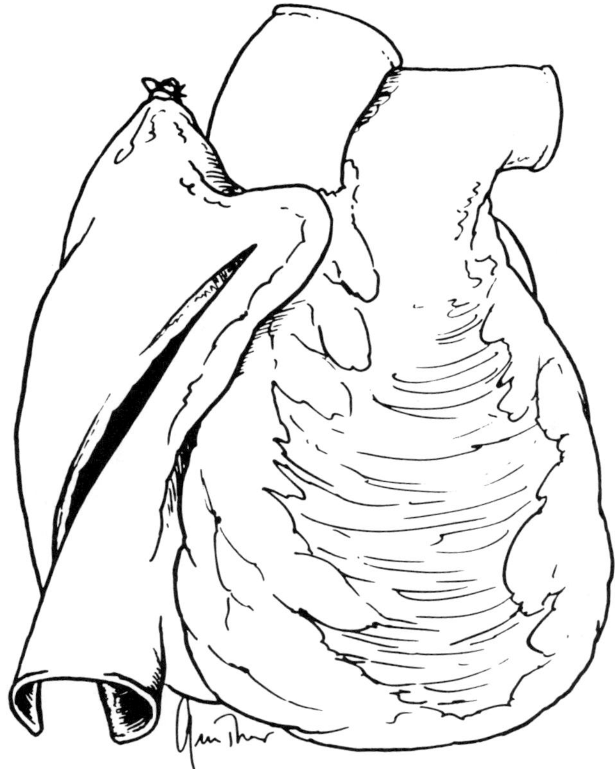

Figure 7: *Completed implantation. Note that the donor right and left pulmonary arteries can be bilaterally fishmouthed to enlarge the pulmonary anastomosis. This large anastomosis may be helpful when there is a large, recipient–donor, pulmonary-artery size discrepancy and to prevent anastomotic stenosis as the infant or child grows.*

pylene (Fig. 8). In most cases, the procedure can be performed without additional cardioplegia—the initial infusion at donor procurement being adequate. The heart is irrigated and bathed with cold topical slush throughout the implantation. If the implantation is prolonged or cardiac activity recurs prematurely, blood cardioplegia is infused via the donor aortic root catheter after deairing.

With completion of the anastomosis, the aortic vent and LV vent are placed on gentle cardiotomy suction, the aortic cross clamp is removed, and the perfusate is slowly warmed to normothermia. Cardiac activity usually returns spontaneously. At normothermia, the

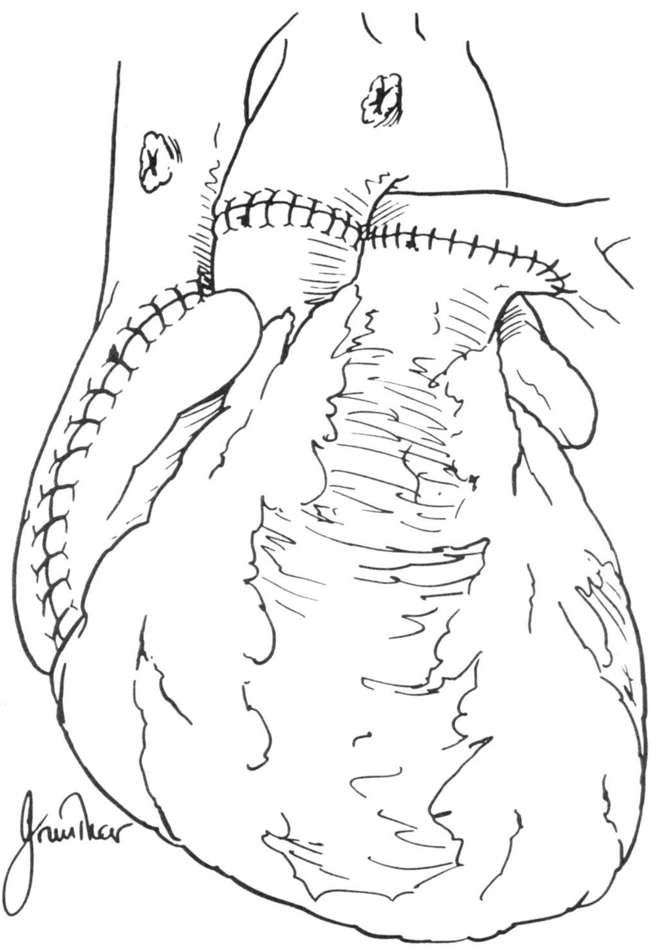

Figure 8: *Completed transplant.*

heart is rested on bypass in the beating, vented mode. Isuprel is begun for cardiac support and with the expectation of early sinus bradycardia, a frequent event in the early posttransplant period. The patient is slowly weaned from cardiopulmonary bypass. Care is taken to avoid bradycardia and cardiac distension. The pulmonary artery pressure is monitored for hypertension and elevated pulmonary vascular resistance (PVR), a common occurrence in patients with chronic cardiomyopathy and certain congenital cardiac lesions. After placement of two atrial and ventricular pacemaker wires and chest drains, the pericardium is closed, plicating the redundant pericardium to obliterate excess space for potential fluid collection. The sternum is closed in a usual fashion.

Operative Immunosuppressive Regimen

Preoperatively, the recipient is given 2–3 mg/kg of cyclosporine and 2 mg/kg Imuran. *Intraoperatively,* Solu-Medrol 10 mg/kg is infused intravenously when the aortic cross clamp is removed. ATGAM (horse antithymacyte globulin) 10 mg/kg in 10 cc/kg D5W is infused over 4 hours starting with cessation of cardiopulmonary bypass (Table 3). *Postoperative* and chronic immunosuppression is discussed in full in Chapter 8. (see Table 2.)

Table 3 Perioperative Immunosuppression

PreOperatively

1. Cyclosporine 3–5 mg/kg P.O.
2. Imuran 2 mg/kg P.O.

Intraoperatively

1. Solumedral 10 mg/kg I.V. (at release of aortic cross clamp)
2. Atgam 10 mg/kg (at cessation of cardiopulmonary bypass)

Special Pediatric Considerations

In general, the operative implantation parallels that in our adult population. Bypass oxygenators, tubing, and cannulae are modified appropriately for size, according to procedures familiar to all pediatric heart centers (Table 4).

Although concerns persist about the ultimate restriction produced by circumferential aortic and pulmonary anastomosis in a growing patient, these problems have not occurred clinically to our knowledge and certainly not in our experience. We have utilized some of the excess ascending aorta to fashion a fish-mouth aortic anastomosis to enlarge the lumen and obviate against later stricture. We have splayed the origins of the left and right pulmonary arteries to fashion an enlarged pulmonary artery anastomosis (Fig. 6) in infants and small children. Although this produces an enlarged anastomotic lumen, care must be taken that excess length of the resulting pulmonary artery does not kink producing a dynamic obstruction.

Table 4 Pediatric Catheters for Cardiopulmonary Bypass

Venous Flow (L/min)	USCL (F)	Pacifico Angled	Riggs (mm)
<0.9	16	16 (3.8 mm)	4
0.9–1.2	20	20 (5.3 mm)	5
1.2–1.6	22	20 (5.3 mm)	5
1.6–1.75	24	24 (5.3 mm)	5
1.7–2.2	28	24 (16.5 mm)	6
2.2–2.8	30	28 (7.45 mm)	6
2.8–3.2	32	28 (7.45 mm)	6
3.2–3.7	34	28 (7.45 mm)	7
>3.7	36	32 (8.0 mm)	7

The above venous cannulae are used in pairs. We prefer the right-angled catheters (Pacifico or Riggs). The catheter sizes are based on manufacture's data and our experience.

Increasingly, pediatric transplantation is performed for underlying congenital heart disease.[4–11] Modification of the procedure is not necessary for morphologic defects resident in the explanted heart. The surgical procedure, however, must address defects in the remnants of the recipient atrial cuffs and great vessels. The most obvious example of this is the surgical modifications for hypoplastic left heart syndrome (HLHS),[12] techniques that are dealt with at length in another chapter.

Transplantation for patients with transposed or malpositioned great vessels has been performed.[10] The recipient aorta is dissected free from surrounding structures, including the pulmonary artery, from the level of the aortic valve to the mid aortic arch. The main pulmonary artery and branches can be dissected free to the pericardial reflections. Using these maneuvers and utilizing the extra length gained from both donor and recipient great vessels, these vessels can be anastomosed without the use of foreign material. There is no reason why even radical techniques such as the Lacompte maneuver,[13] routinely utilized in arterial switch procedures, could not be utilized. In our only experience in transplanting a patient with transposed great vessels, the aortic anastomosis was accomplished to the underside of the proximal aortic arch, and the pulmonary anastomosis was accomplished at the bifurcation of the recipient pulmonary artery.

Atrial septal defects of the recipient atrial septum can be easily repaired with extraordinary exposure after removal of the old ventricular mass. Complex abnormalities of the atrium and venous return can be managed with pericardial atrial baffles. It would seem that virtually all such defects can be repaired during the transplant procedure. It is essential that the techniques for adapting the specific congenital cardiac defect to the transplant procedure be evaluated and worked out in advance.

Myocardial Protection of the Pediatric Heart

Myocardial protection for the donor heart has, in general, reflected the protection utilized during other open heart procedures. Myocardial protection during cardiac operations has been extensively researched in the adult population and the use of crystalloid or blood cardioplegia is now the method of choice in adult cardiac surgery. However, the efficacy of cardioplegia to protect the immature myocardium in cardiac operations involving children, infants, and newborns is still controversial.[14–16]

The controversy is largely caused by the lack of studies on myocardial protection that take into account the different structure, function, and metabolism of the immature myocardium. Compared with the adult heart, the immature myocardium has smaller myocytes, reduced density of contractile units, fewer organized fibers, reduced numbers of mitochondria, and more rudimentary sarcoplasmic reticulum.[17–19]

Probably as a consequence of the different structure, the immature myocardium is able to develop less tension[20] and is less compliant than the adult myocardium.[21]

Metabolic studies have recently delineated substantial differences between adult and mature myocardium. The immature myocardium uses preferentially anaerobic glycolysis and has the capability of reducing the waste of ATP products. In addition, it is able to rebuild ATP more rapidly by three mechanisms: increased mitochondrial ATP, increased adenine nucleotide translocase, and 5′-nucleotidasis.[22–24] On the other hand, the reduced myofibrilla ATPase activity may explain why the immature myocardium is able to produce less active tension than the adult heart.[25] Finally, optimal levels of extracellular calcium concentrations are critical in the pediatric population to maintain adequate inotropism.[26,27] The immature myocardium, in fact, is unable to sequester calcium to the same extent as the mature myocardium, presumably due to its undeveloped sarcoplasmic reticulum.

Although structural, functional, and metabolic differences between adult and immature heart are now well established, only a limited number of experimental and clinical studies have compared their specific responses to ischemia. The experimental evidence would indicate that the neonatal heart has greater tolerance to ischemia than the more mature myocardium,[28,29] probably due to its increased capability to utilize the anaerobic glycolytic pathway and its ability to rebuild ATP more rapidly. This greater resistance to ischemia, however, seems to disappear within 6 to 8 weeks after birth. In a recent study, Watanabe et al.[31] confirmed that during ischemia, the neonatal guinea pig myocardium maintained higher levels of high-energy phosphate compounds compared with the adult guinea pig myocardium. In addition, the authors investigated factors inducing contracture[30] (increased resting tension) during ischemia. Contracture, a sensitive index of cell damage, occurred only in the immature myocardium and only after infusion of crystalloid cardioplegia. This disturbing finding would indicate that crystalloid cardioplegia induced contracture in the immature heart in spite of the fact that the immature myocardium was metabolically more resistant to ischemia. In another study[31] comparing the different mechanical responses to cardioplegic solution shown by the neonatal and the adult guinea pig myocardium, the same authors demonstrated that the differences were not due to changes of the membrane potential. They suggested that the contracture seen in the ischemic immature heart exposed to cardioplegia was due to disruption of the intracellular calcium regulation and concluded that further studies should address the role of calcium metabolism during ischemia in the immature heart. The composition of cardioplegic solutions utilized to protect the mature myocardium should probably take into account the role of calcium during ischemia.

Nevertheless, other investigators[32–34] have shown that cardioplegia is more effective than hypothermia alone in preserving contractility and compliance of the immature myocardium. The systolic function of isolated pig hearts following 2 hours of ischemic arrest was studied by Corno et al.[35] Good systolic function was maintained after topical cooling alone (8–10°C), with crystalloid cardioplegia, and blood cardioplegia. However, in this study, the optimal recovery was obtained in hearts protected with cold-blood cardioplegia containing 16 mmEq/L of potassium and 1.2 mEq/L calcium. Finally, in a recent study comparing single-dose versus multiple-dose crystalloid cardioplegia in the newborn rabbit (from birth to 2 days of age), Sawa et al.[36] demonstrated that the newborn myocardium receiving a single dose of cold cardioplegia was well preserved during 120 min of ischemia without showing significant mitochondrial damage and cellular study, multiple doses of crystalloid cardioplegia produced significant mitochondrial damage with cellular edema. The authors concluded that multiple doses in the newborn myocardium damaged the endothelial cells of the microvasculature by washing out the red cells and proteins and increased microvasculature permeability.

Only a limited number of clinical studies are currently available on myocardial protection in pediatric cardiac surgery. Bull et al.[13] showed that in their experience the use of cardioplegia did not appear to provide a substantial degree of protection and suggested that in their patients there was direct correlation between cytochemical evidence of myocardial deterioration and patient's death. Sawa et al.[36] showed significant mitochondrial injury in infants under 3 months of age undergoing cardiac repair and were unable to demonstrate significant myocardial protection by cold crystalloid cardioplegia in these patients. Finally, in a study on blood cardioplegia, Del Nido showed no advantages of using blood cardioplegia for myocardial protection during repair of tetralogy of Fallot.

In conclusion, optimal myocardial protection in pediatric population is not established. When the experimental and clinical evidence is applied to cardiac transplantation in children, it seems reasonable to conclude that a combination of topical hypothermia and cold, single-dose, cardioplegia solution should be used to protect the donor heart. However, although most centers accept a total ischemia time of approximately 4 hours in adults, we believe that in-house retrieval should be used for newborn and infant transplantation. Additional protection can be obtained during the recipient operation by the technique of deep hypothermia and low flow, or circulatory arrest in patients less than 10 kg. In older children, in whom often adult-size hearts are implanted, a period of total ischemia similar to the one accepted in adults is usually well tolerated. In children less than 10 years of age, no clear data are available on the safety of total ischemia time. In this age group, it would be reasonable to prefer locally procured hearts and to maintain ischemia time less than 100 min.

Postoperative Care

The early postoperative care varies only slightly from the management of any other patient recovering after cardiopulmonary bypass. In general, most complications are secondary to the hemodynamics of the postbypass heart and not related to rejection. It is essential to manage the posttransplant patient and problems as they develop in the same systematic approach utilized in the nontransplant bypass patient. Problems such as bleeding, tamponade, arrhythmias, low cardiac output, and respiratory failure occur in the transplant child and must be evaluated and treated as if they are not secondary to rejection.

Most patients will hemodynamically recover quickly from transplantation and respond to minimal inotropic support. Initially following transplantation, the recipient is encumbered with intubation and mechanical ventilation, multiple central lines (CVP and pulmonary artery), and at least one inotrope—isoproterenol. All efforts are made to aggressively wean the patient from this support within the first 24 hours. This is usually passable in the routine transplant child. Not only does removing all invasive paraphernalia markedly reduce the risk of nosocomial infection in the immunosuppressed patient, but it also allows the child to become mobile, exercise, and immediately begin countering the catabolic effects of immunosuppressive steroids. It is also our impression that an early mobilization and exercise program stimulates an increased heart rate, obviating the need for extended chronotropic support and allowing earlier removal of the temporary pacing wires.

Rejection is usually not the etiology of early postoperative hemodynamic failure. Hyperacute rejection is rarely seen. When it occurs, it is manifested with immediate severe cardiac failure occurring as soon as circulation is restored in the operating room. The more common acute rejection that we more routinely experience in the immunosuppressed recipient manifests itself much later—days to weeks—after transplantation, and usually presents with a positive biopsy, not clinical symptoms. The evaluation of rejection and its treatment is reviewed in Chapters 8 and 11.

Hemodynamic complications are the consequence of: (1) the depressed myocardium following cardioplegic arrest and bypass, (2) the denervated transplanted heart, and (3) the consequences of pulmonary vascular resistance.

The transplanted heart usually maintains an adequate contractile state despite prolonged cold arrest for up to 4 hours. It is, however, noncompliant and often exhibits an inability to increasing stroke volume and hence cardiac output. Coupled with a slow rate secondary to denervation and sinoatrial node dysfunction, the transplanted heart may be unable to respond appropriately with increased output. The stiff transplanted heart thus requires a high filling pressure to maximize stroke work. The slow sinus or nodal rate often seen after transplantation can be managed with isoproterenol and atrial pacing. Inotropic agents should be used judiciously, but whenever indicated.

Elevated *pulmonary vascular resistance* and pulmonary hypertension secondary to chronic cardiomyopathy or congenital heart disease are contraindications when severe (PVR >6-8 woods u). When mild, pulmonary vascular resistance is not a contraindication to transplantation, but is still of concern. After cardiopulmonary bypass and its inherent vascular endothelial damage, pulmonary vascular resistance may be transiently greater than prebypass, as well as more difficult to manage. In addition, left heart failure and decreased compliance necessitate a high left ventricular end-diastolic pressure. Both of these events result in an elevation of pulmonary artery pressure. The transplanted heart, with its "normal" right ventricle, may not be prepared for this increased afterload and indeed, may function less well in the presence of pulmonary hypertension than the discarded recipient right ventricle. All efforts, then, must be made, prior to weaning from bypass and in the early postoperative period, to reduce the left ventricular end-diastolic pressure, to reduce pulmonary vascular resistance, and hence, pulmonary arterial pressure.

All patients are managed intraoperatively and in the early postoperative period with a pulmonary artery catheter to aid in monitoring pulmonary arterial pressure, cardiac output, and pulmonary vascular resistance. Routinely, an isoproterenol infusion is begun prior to weaning from bypass. Not only does this promote pulmonary vasodilatation, but it is also the inotropic agent of choice because of its chronotropic effect on the slow heart. In addition, when pulmonary vascular resistance is a concern preoperatively (PVR > 3–4 woods u), we will often begin an amrinone infusion preoperatively and continue it throughout bypass and the early postoperative period.

In the face of severe right heart failure and an elevated pulmonary vascular resistance and pulmonary hypertensive crisis, we employ a "fire drill" identical to that used for congenital heart cases with pulmonary hypertension. It is essential, that such a protocol be established to manage the posttransplant patient with pulmonary hypertensive crisis. At our institution, this includes controlled mechanical ventilation with sedation and paralysis of the patient. The patient is hyperventilated with an FIO_2 of 100% inducing a hypocarbia (PCO_2 = 25–30 mm Hg) and mild respiratory alkalosis. Drug stimulation of pulmonary vasodilatation utilized nitroglycerin, nitroprusside, prostaglandin (PGE_2), and tolazouline. These drugs can be infused separately or in combination through a right atrial or central pulmonary artery line.

Frequently, the patient with a severe pulmonary hypertensive crisis requires inotropic support as well. All efforts should be made to avoid drugs that stimulate pulmonary vascular tone, relying instead on drugs such as amrinone, low-dose dopamine, dolbutamine, and especially isoproterenol. When more potent inotropes such as epinephrine, levophed, and high-dose dopamine are required, they should be infused through the left atrial line to avoid the pulmonary circuit, and their pulmonary vasoconstrictive effect should be aggressively countered with a right-sided infusion of a pulmonary vasodilator.

With this protocol, mild to severe pulmonary vascular resistance elevation can usually be managed, the support being judiciously reduced after 2–3 days as the pulmonary vascular resistance falls and the transplanted heart stabilizes.

References

1. McGoon DC: Closure of patent ductus during open heart surgery. Nurs Forum 1964, 48:458.
2. Steinson EB, Dong E, Schraeder JS, et al: Initial clinical experience with heart transplantation. Am J Cardiol 1968, 22:791.
3. Cooley DA, Bloodwell RD, Hallman GL, et al: Cardiac transplantation: General considerations and results. Ann Surg 1969, 169:892.
4. Penkoske PA, Rowe RD, Freedom RM, et al: The future of heart and heart–lung transplantation in children. Heart Transplant 1984, 3:233.
5. Pennington DG, Sarafian J, Swarts M: Heart transplantation in children. Heart Transplant 1985, IV:441.
6. Addonizio LJ, Rose EA: Cardiac transplantation in children and adolescents. J Pediatr 1987, 111:1034.
7. Dunn JM, Cavarocchi NC, Balsara RK, et al: Pediatric heart transplantation at St. Christopher's Hospital for Children. Heart Transplant 1987, 6:334.
8. Kaye MP: The registry of the international society of heart transplantation: Fourth report—1987. Heart Transplant 1987, 6:63.
9. Starnes VA, Stinson E, Oyer P, et al: Cardiac transplantation in children and adolescents. Circulation 76(Suppl V) 1987:V43.
10. Harjula ALJ, Heikkila LJ, Nieminen MS, et al: Heart transplantation in repaired transposition of the great arteries. Ann Thorac Surg 1988, 46: 611.

11. Macoviak J, Baldwin JC, Ginsburg R, et al: Orthotopic cardiac transplantation for univentricular heart. Ann Thorac Surg 1988, 45:85.
12. Bailey LL, Assand AN, Trimm RF, et al: Orthotopic transplantation during early infancy as therapy for incurable congenital heart disease. Ann Surg 1988, 208:279.
13. Bical D, Hazan E, Lecompte Y, et al: Anatomic correction of transposition of the great arteries with ventricular septal defect: Results in 50 patients. Circulation 1984, 70:891.
14. Kirklin JK, Blackstone EH, Kirklin JW, et al: Intracardiac surgery in infants under age 3 months: Incremental risk factors for hospital morality. Am J Cardiol 1981, 48:500.
15. Bull C, Cooper J, Stark J: Cardioplegic protection of the child's heart. J Thorac Cardiovasc Surg 1984, 88:287.
16. Watanabe H, Yokosawa T, Eguchi S, et al: Functional and metabolic protection of the neonatal myocardium from ischemia. J Thorac Cardiovasc Surg 1989, 97:50.
17. Rudolph AM, Heymann MA: Fetal and neonatal circulation and respiration. Annu Rev Physiol 1974, 36:187.
18. Sheldon CA, Friedman WF, Sylers HD: Scanning electron microscopy of fetal and neonatal lamb cardiac cells. J Mol Cell Cardiol 1976, 8:853.
19. Maylie JG: Excitation-contraction coupling in neonatal and adult myocardium of cat. Am J Physiol 1982, 242:H834.
20. Friedman WF: The intrinsic physiologic properties of the developing heart. Prog Cardiovasc Dis 1972, 15:87.
21. Romero T, Friedman WF: Limited left ventricular response to volume overload in the neonatal period: A comparative study with the adult animal. Pediatr Res 1979, 13:910.
22. Dawes GS, Mott JC, Shelley HJ: The importance of cardiac glycogen for the maintenance of life in foetal lambs and newborn animals during anoxia. J Physiol 1959, 146:516.
23. Young HH, Shimizu T, Nishioka K, et al: Effect of hypoxia and reoxygenation on mitochondrial function in neonatal myocardium. Am J Physiol 1983, 245:998.
24. Wechsler AS, Abd-Elfattah As, Murphy CE, et al: Myocardial protection. J Cardiac Surg 1986, 3:271.
25. Nakanishi T, Jarmakani JM: Developmental changes in myocardial mechanical function and subcellular organelles. Am J Physiol 1984, 246: H615.
26. Seguchi M, Harding JA, Jarmakani JM: Developmental change in the function of sarcoplasmic reticulum. J Mol Cell Cardiol 1986, 18:189.
27. Nishioka K, Nakanishi T, George BL, et al: The effect of calcium on the inotropy of catecholamine and paired electrical stimulation in the newborn and adult myocardium. J Mol Cell Cardiol 1981, 13:511.
28. Starnes VA, Hammon JW Jr: The influence of acute global ischemia on left ventricular compliance in the adult and immature dog. J Surg Res 1981, 30:281.
29. Bove EL, Stammers AH: Recovery of left ventricular function after hypo-

thermic global ischemia: Age-related differences in the isolated working rabbit heart. J Thorac Cardiovasc Surg 1986, 91:115.
30. Hearse DJ, Glarlick BP, Humphrey SM: Ischemic contracture of the myocardium. Mechanisms and prevention. Am J Cardiol 1977, 39:986.
31. Watanabe H, Yokosawa T, Eguchi S, et al: Difference in the mechanical response to a cardioplegic solution observed between the neonatal and the adult guinea pig myocardium. J Thorac Cardiovasc Surg 1989, 97:59.
32. Wisman CB, Waldhausen JA, Pierce WS, et al: Preservation of myocardial high-energy phosphates during ischemia in the isolated perfused neonatal pig heart: A comparison of hypothermic potassium cardioplegia with hypothermia alone. Surg Forum 1982, 33:315.
33. Bove EL, Stammers AH, Gallagher KP: Protection of the neonatal myocardium during hypothermic ischemia: Effect of cardioplegia on left ventricular function in the rabbit. J Thorac Cardiovasc Surg 1987, 94:115.
34. Ganzel BL, Gott JP, Katzmark S, et al: Hemodynamic effects of surface cooling-induced hypothermia on immature pigs with ventricular septal defects. Surgery 1985, 98:516.
35. Corno AF, Bethencourt DM, Laks H, et al: Myocardial protection in the neonatal heart: A comparison of topical hypothermia and crystalloid and blood cardioplegic solutions. J Thorac Cardiovasc Surg 1987, 93:163.
36. Sawa Y, Matsuda H, Shimazaki Y, et al: Ultrastructural assessment of the infant myocardium receiving crystalloid cardioplegia. Circulation 1987, 76(Suppl V):V141.

Chapter 7

Infant Orthotopic Cardiac Transplantation

Constantine Mavroudis

Introduction

Infant orthotopic cardiac transplantation (OCT) has been shown to be an effective short-term treatment for conventionally untreatable forms of congenital heart disease.[1–6] These advances, however, have come only recently compared with the successes of adult orthotopic cardiac transplantation. Reasons for this delay can be attributed to: a limited donor pool, lack of convincing data concerning myocardial preservation in the newborn infant, uncertainty of long-term immunosuppression and its consequences, and philosophical objections. Recent advances with animal experimentation,[7–10] improvements with extended neonatal cardiopulmonary bypass,[11] and facility with cyclosporine immunosuppression[12–14] have allowed the implementation of infant orthotopic cardiac transplant centers to evaluate the short- and long-term effects of OCT, immunosuppression, and quality of life.

Patients and Methods

Between June 1986 and October 1988, we evaluated 22 infants who were candidates for OCT. Twenty had hypoplastic left heart syndrome (HLHS), one had endocardial fibroelastosis with severe aortic stenosis, and one had ischemic cardiomyopathy because of undiagnosed anomalous pulmonary artery origin of the left main coronary

From *Heart Transplantation in Children*, edited by Jeffrey M. Dunn, M.D. and Richard M. Donner, M.D.

artery (ACA). Staged orthoterminal correction[15] was not employed because of early, high-mortality rates and unsatisfactory results shown in many centers.[16] More recently, however, the results of stages orthoterminal correction have been improving, and this method of treatment may prove to be a suitable alternative therapy when donor hearts are not available. Patients were screened by physicians and trained social workers to determine their ability to comply with treatment regimens. All of our patients, except one, originated from our usual referral pattern based on a population of 2.8 million people, with a rate of 14 live births per thousand population.

All families received initial counseling that emphasized the experimental nature of the operation. As more transplants were performed, we were able to provide more objective data to families concerning their posttransplant duties and responsibilities. As a result of this family education program, 11 families refused the treatment regimen (2 because of associated anomalies and 9 for personal reasons, Table 1). Another 11 families accepted the treatment protocol. Of these patients, 3 died before transplantation could be accomplished (Table 2). The other 8 infants (7 with HLHS and 1 with ACA) underwent OCT.

All organ donors were fully evaluated by local physicians with neurologic and cardiologic consultation before transport to our institution. Brain death was diagnosed by a combination of findings that included electroencephalogram, physical examination, and blood flow studies. Cardiac function was evaluated by electrocardiogram, echocardiogram, and vital signs (Table 3). Other evaluation included organ size, body mass, standard chest roentgenogram, ABO blood type compatibility, and absence of systemic or infectious disease.

We initially based donor–recipient size matchup on a donor size variance of ± 1,000 gm referable to the recipient. The paucity of donors, however, forced us to examine other measures of size compatibility that we discovered when comparing donor–recipient chest roentgenographs. We were thus able to use larger donors as long as the cardiac silhouettes on standard size roentgenographs[5] were comparable (Fig. 1, Table 4). Because in-house retrieval was used for all transplants, brain-dead organ donors were transported to our institution, where all studies were confirmed. Multiple organ procurement was practiced at our institution by participating transplant teams. Donor heart dissection proceeded with careful preservation of the entire aortic arch well downstream to the ductus arteriosus into the left chest

Table 1 Clinical and Social Characteristics of Infants and Families Who Refused Transplants

	Disease	Associated Anomalies	Parental Characteristics	Reasons for Refusal
Parent #1	Endocardial fibroelactosis aortic atresia	None	Married college students with parental support	Worried about child's future, would try again for normal child
Parent #2	HLHS	Cleft lip and others	Stable relationship, six normal children	Child had too many problems to overcome
Parent #3	HLHS	None	Unmarried young couple	Worried about responsibility of child care
Parent #4	HLHS	None	Married parents, stable relationship, career Army	Worried about child's future, would try again for normal child
Parent #5	HLHS	Trisomy #13, other problems	Stable relationship	Parents agreed that child was not a candidate for OCT
Patient #6	HLHS	None	Stable relationship	Worried about child's future, would try again for normal child
Patient #7	HLHS	None	Young (under 16 years of age) unmarried couple	Worried about responsibility of child care
Patient #8	HLHS	None	Young couple, limited means and transportation	Worried about responsibility of child care
Patient #9	Endocardial fibroelastosis Coarctation	None	Married/stable, 3 "healthy" children at home	Neurologic complications, developed seizures
Patient #10	HLHS	None	Unmarried young parents (High School)	Worried about experimental nature of transplant
Patient #11	HLHS	None	Married/stable, first child	Would try again for healthy child

HLHS = hypoplastic left heart syndrome; OCT = orthotopic cardiac transplantation. Augmented and reproduced with permission from Mavroudis et al.[5]

Table 2 Clinical and Social Characteristics of Infants and Families Who Wanted Transplant But Was Not Done

	Disease	Size (kg)	Parental Characteristics	Outcome
Parent #1	HLHS	4.1	Stable relationship, 7 normal children	Child died 6 hours after diagnosis
Parent #2	HLHS	3.3	Stable relationship, 1 child from prior marriage	Baby developed neurologic complications, was allowed to die after 60 days on transplant donor network
Parent #3	HLHS	2.9	Stable relationship, no previous children	Patient allowed to die after congenital CMV was discovered

CMV = cytomegalic virus infection; HLHS = hypoplastic left heart syndrome; reproduced with permission from Mavroudis et al.[5]

Table 3 Clinical Characteristics of Donors

	Reason for Brain Death	Echo Percent Fiber Shortening (%)	Cardiotonic Drugs at Transplantation	State Origin of Donor
Donor #1	Perinatal Asphyxiation	39	None	Mass.
Donor #2	SIDS	32	None	Idaho
Donor #3	SIDS/Aspiration	38	None	Calif.
Donor #4	Motor Vehicle Accident	27	Dopamine 5 mic/kg/min	Mich.
Donor #5	SIDS	47	None	Tenn.
Donor #6	Shaken Baby Syndrome	21–24	Dopamine 5 mic/kg/min	Tenn.
Donor #7	Hydrocephalus Intraventricular bleed	33	None	Ohio
Donor #8	Ischemic Brain Injury	29	Dopamine 20 mic/kg/min	Missouri

SIDS = sudden infant death syndrome; augmented and reproduced with permission from Mavroudis et al.[5]

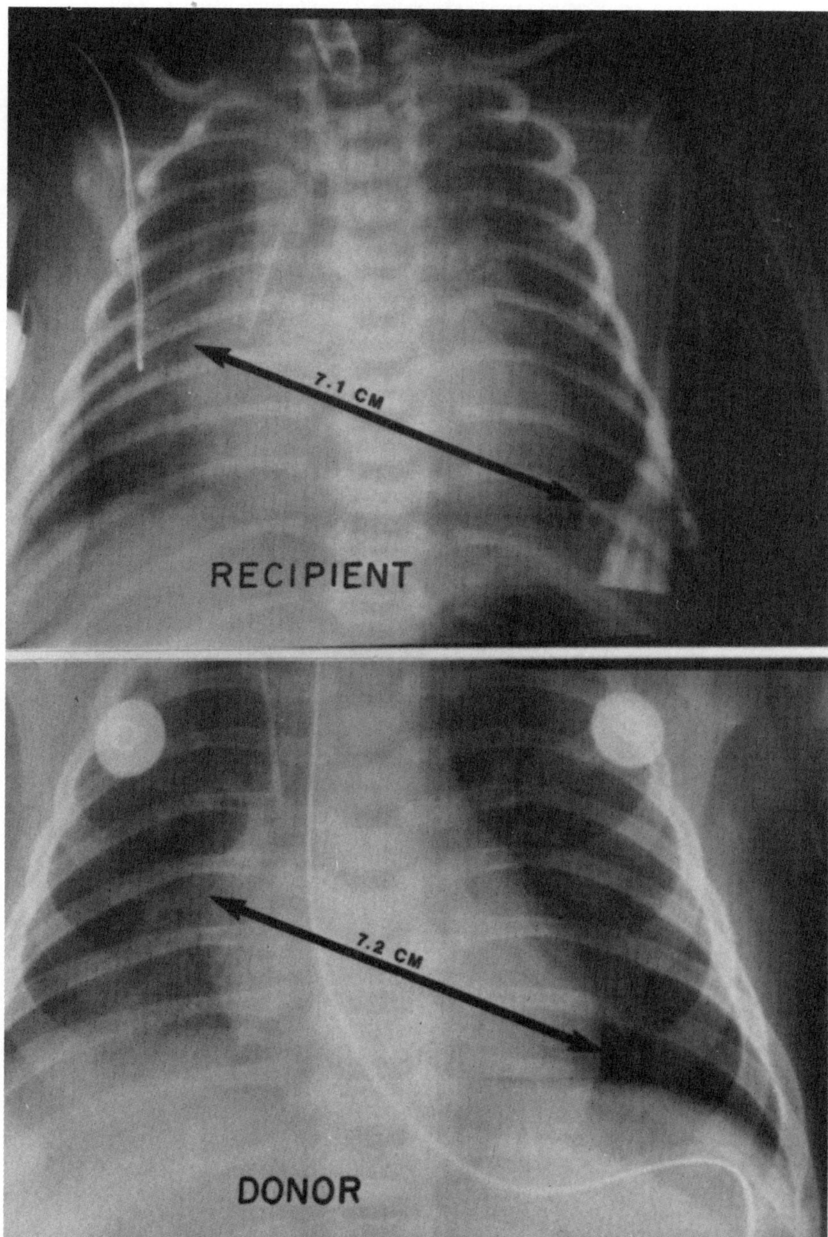

Figure 1: *Recipient and donor A-P chest roentgenographs taken by standard portable equipment with a 36-inch focal distance. Arrows show the direction (mid-right atrium to apex of the heart) and magnitude of measurements. When donor–recipient weight variance was greater than 1,000 gm, this method of size evaluation proved helpful (Table 3). Reproduced with permission from Mavroudis et al.*[5]

Table 4 Donor–Recipient Match

	Body Mass (kg)	Age at Operation	Blood Type	Crossmatch	HLA Match	CXR* Cardiac Size (cm)
Patient #1	2.7	23 days	O+	Neg	0/6	7.0
Donor #1	3.0	7 days	O+			6.4
Patient #2	6.8	11 months	B+	Neg	0/6	12.0
Donor #2	6.5	5 months	O+			6.5
Patient #3	2.2	8 days	A+	Neg	0/6	6.2
Donor #3	3.6	4 days	O−			5.5
Patient #4	3.9	9 days	O−	Neg	1/6	7.1
Donor #4	6.5	9 weeks	O−			7.2
Patient #5	3.3	13 days	A+	Neg	0/6	7.1
Donor #5	4.8	4 months	A+			7.2
Patient #6	3.5	5 days	A+	Neg	0/6	7.2
Donor #6	4.8	3 months	O+			6.2
Patient #7	3.3	22 days	B+	Neg	0/6	6.3
Donor #7	4.0	6 days	O+			5.5
Patient #8	3.5	26 days	O−	Neg	1/6	9.2
Donor #8	3.9	2 days	O+			6.4

*Roentgenographs performed by standard portable equipment with a 36-inch focal distance; Augmented and reproduced with permission from Mavroudis et al.[5]

cavity. In an adjacent operating room, the recipient was placed on cardiopulmonary bypass and cooled to 15°C in preparation for circulatory arrest and OCT. The donor heart was then excised after cardioplegic arrest and transferred to the recipient's room, where the patent foramen ovale was closed and the aortic arch trimmed to size for aortic reconstruction.

The operative procedure was based on standard techniques for OCT.[3,17] Profound hypothermia and circulatory arrest was used in seven neonates with HLHS, and moderate hypothermia with bicaval cannulation and continuous cardiopulmonary bypass was used for an 11-month old infant with ACA (Table 5). Aortic reconstruction in the neonatal HLHS group was dependent on the size of the ascending aorta. Five patients with hypoplastic ascending aorta underwent extensive arch reconstruction (Figs. 2–6), and two others with adequately sized ascending aorta underwent simple, aortic, end-to-end anastomosis below the recipient innominate artery. Polydioxanone 5-0 and 6-0 suture was used for the anastomoses.

Table 5 Operative Characteristics

	Disease	Bypass Technique	Arch Reconstruction	Arrest Time	Outcome
Patient #1	HLHS	Deep hypothermia in circulatory arrest	No	48 min	A & W
Patient #2	ACA	Moderate hypothermia and bicaval cannulation continuous bypass	No	N/A	A & W
Patient #3	HLHS	Deep hypothermia circulatory arrest	Yes	50 min	Died
Patient #4	HLHS	Deep hypothermia circulatory arrest	No	42 min	A & W
Patient #5	HLHS	Deep hypothermia circulatory arrest	Yes	48 min	A & W
Patient #6	HLHS	Deep hypothermia circulatory arrest	Yes	52 min	Died
Patient #7	HLHS	Deep hypothermia circulatory arrest	Yes	63 min, 34 min	Died
Patient #8	HLHS	Deep hypothermia circulatory arrest	Yes	48 min	A & W

HLHS = hypoplastic left heart syndrome; Augmented and reproduced with permission from Mavroudis et al.[5]

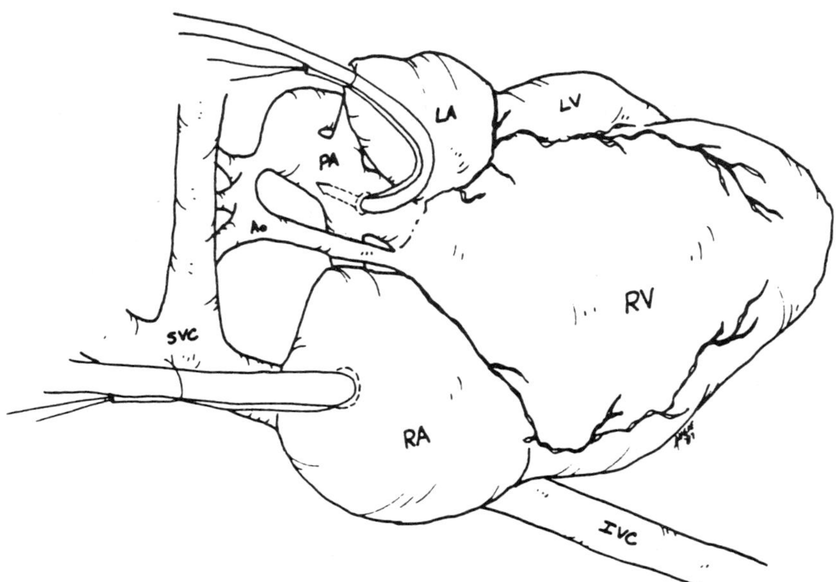

Figure 2: *Diagrammatic drawing showing pertinent anatomical landmarks of a typical patient with Type IA[1-4] hypoplastic left heart syndrome. Systemic flow is by pulmonary artery cannulation (through the ductus arteriosus) and venous return by single atrial cannulation. Reproduced with permission from Mavroudis et al.[5]*

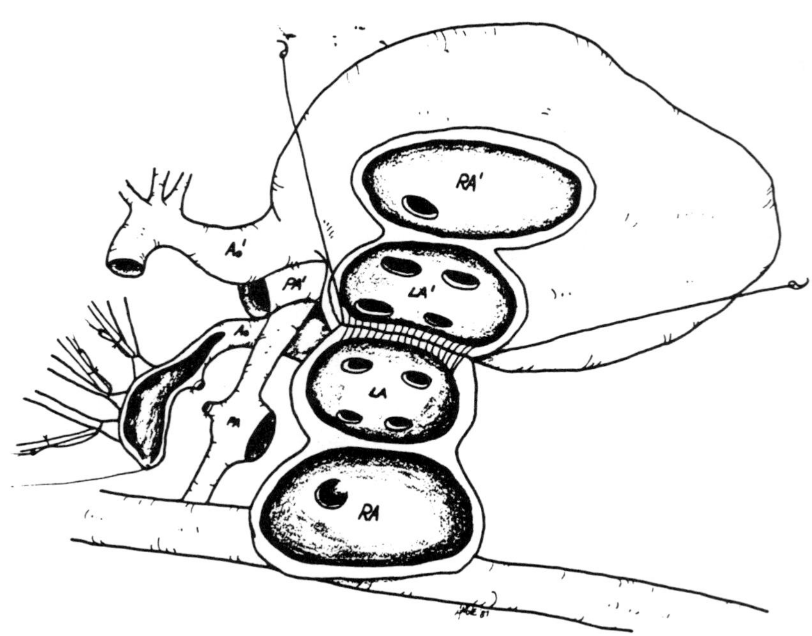

Figure 3: *Diagrammatic drawing showing the result of deep hypothermia, circulatory arrest, removal of the hypoplastic heart, longitudinal aortic arch incision downstream to the coarctation, and ligated ductus arteriosus. The left atrial suture line is shown as the first step towards graft implantation. Reproduced with permission from Mavroudis et al.*[5]

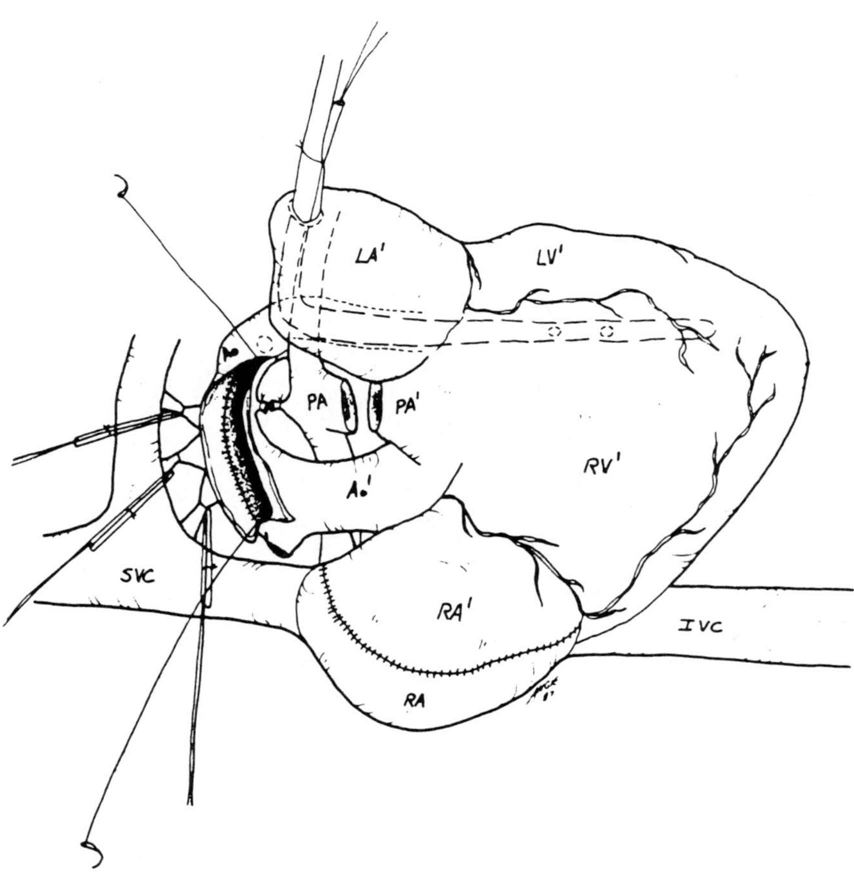

Figure 4: *Diagrammatic drawing showing completed atrial anastomoses. A left ventricular catheter (10F) is placed (via left atrium) to instill cold saline (4°C) for myocardial protection and air removal. Initiation of the aortic arch reconstruction is depicted. The donor innominate artery stump is preserved for aortic cannulation following aortic arch reconstruction. Standard abbreviations are used to denote recipient and donor (with prime, i.e. Ao') structures. Reproduced with permission from Mavroudis et al.*[5]

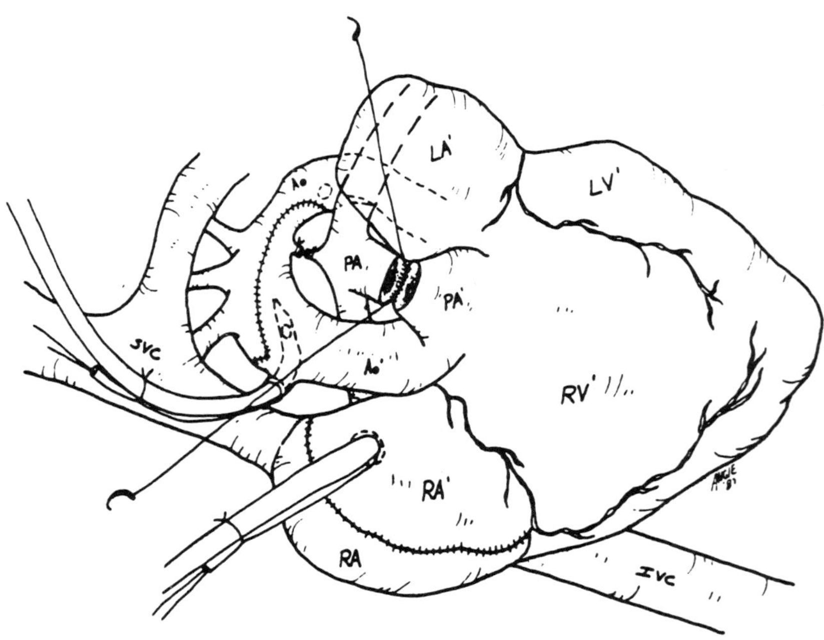

Figure 5: *Diagrammatic drawing showing completed atrial anastomoses, aortic arch reconstruction and partial pulmonary artery suture line. Aortic cannulation (via the donor innominate artery stump) and right atrial cannulation have been accomplished followed by cavitary air evacuation, cardiopulmonary bypass, and rewarming. Standard abbreviations are used to denote recipient and donor (with prime, i.e. Ao') structures. Reproduced with permission from Mavroudis et al.*[5]

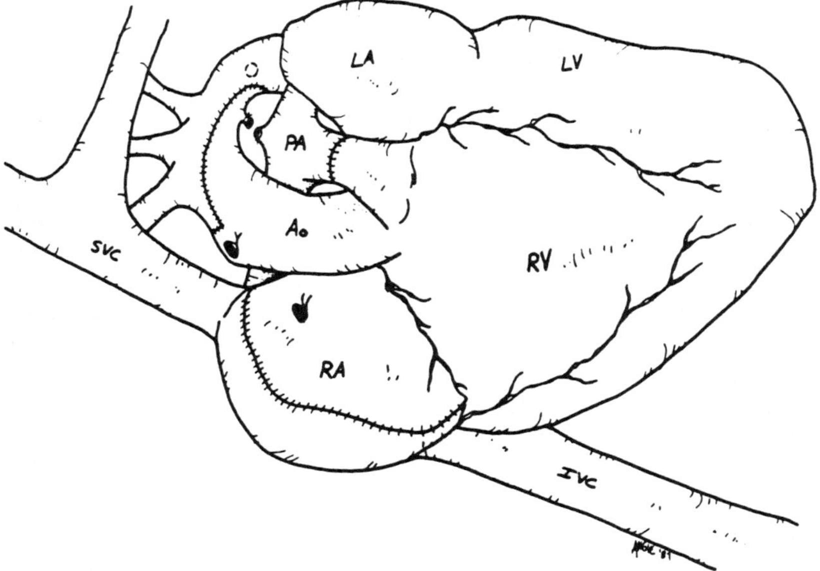

Figure 6: *Diagrammatic drawing of completed graft implantation. If size discrepancy or graft swelling intervenes, a silastic skin patch*[20] *can be applied with secondary closure after swelling subsides. Standard abbreviations are used to denote recipient and donor (with prime, i.e. Ao') structures. Reproduced with permission from Mavroudis et al.*[5]

Immunosuppression and Monocyte–Lymphocyte Cell Cycle Analysis

The initial immunosuppression drug regimen consisted of cyclosporine 0.33 mg/kg/day by continuous intravenous infusion to achieve a whole blood level between 800 and 1,200 ng/mL early in the series, which was amended to 400 to 800 ng/mL later in the series, azathioprine 0.5 mg/kg/day, and methylprednisolone 0.5 mg/kg every 6 hours. When tolerated, oral doses were adjusted to: cyclosporin 20–25 mg/kg/day in two to three doses to achieve the aforementioned whole blood levels, azathioprine 1 mg/kg/day, and prednisone 0.25 mg/kg/day. Because we decided against myocardiac biopsies, the optimal method for diagnosis of graft rejection was to be determined by this study. We prospectively evaluated: (a) clinical examination based on infant activity, feeding habits, and nursing personnel observations; (b) monocyte and lymphocyte replicative cycle kinetics; (c) electrocardiography; (d) echocardiography; and (e) myocardial enzyme analysis.

Determination of monocyte and lymphocyte replicative cycle kinetics was chosen as a possible indicator of allograft rejection. Enumeration of lymphocyte transferrin and interleukin 2 (IL-2) expression has been shown to correlate with cellular activation.[18–20] Flow cytometric measurement of the expression of these activation markers has been utilized as an aid in the diagnosis of cardiac allograft rejection.[21,22] Because the expression of transferrin and IL-2 receptors indicates that the lymphocyte is entering the replicative cycle, we attempted to correlate the phases of the cell cycle with allograft rejection.

The distribution of monocytes or lymphocytes within the replicative cycle was determined by flow microfluorometry, using a modification of the technique described by Braylan and associates.[23] Briefly, mononuclear cells were separated from whole blood by density centrifugation. Approximately 500,000 cells were then stained with fluoresceinisothiocyanate (FITC) conjugated monocyte-2 antibody (Coulter Laboratories, Hialeah, Fla.) The FITC conjugated monocyte-2 antibody specifically stains monocytes and emits green fluorescence, thus permitting the differential analysis of monocytes and lymphocytes. The cell preparation was fixed in 70% ethanol at 4° C to facilitate nuclear staining. The fixed cells were then treated at room temperature for 30 min with 1 mg of RNAse (Sigma Chemicals, St. Louis, Mo.), followed by the addition of propridium iodide (6 μg). Five thousand to 10,000 cells were simultaneously analyzed for surface phenotype (monocyte-2) and DNA content on an Ortho Cytofluorograph IIs flow cytometer (Ortho Diagnostics, Westwood, Mass.). The percentage of cells within the G_0/G_1, S, and G_2/M phases of the replicative cycles was selectively determined on monocyte-2 stained monocyte and unstained lymphocytes. Normal percentages of lymphocytes and monocytes in S and G_2/M phases were determined from 15 measurements when no rejection was clinically apparent. The mean normal values were 2.87; a high index of suspicion was generated when the value exceeded two standard deviations above the normal mean.

Results

Five of the 8 infants survived (63%) and are presently at home, following the drug regimens, and achieving normal growth and developmental milestones. One of the deaths occurred in a neonate with HLHS (ascending aortic hypoplasia and coarctation) and was due to donor heart dysfunction, size discrepancy, and probable coronary air emboli. At the time of implantation, the heart, from a donor resuscitated after sudden infant death, was distended with a rate of only 85 beats/min. OCT and aortic arch reconstruction proceeded without incident, but was complicated by coronary air embolism, ventricular swelling, and ventricular dysfunction. A silicone rubber skin patch[24] was used to maximize the intrathoracic space, but the baby died a few hours later. The second death occurred 2 months after successful OCT and aortic arch reconstruction from unsuspected severe rejection. He was placed on emergency extracorporeal membrane oxygenation but died the following day of heart failure. Postmortem findings confirmed severe cardiac rejection. The third death occurred due to excessive bleeding at the aortic anastomotic site adjacent to the recipient ductal tissue. Attempts at repair resulted in prolonged myocardial ischemia and eventual intraoperative death.

Major complications occurred in three of the remaining five survivors. The first baby (HLHS) sustained a cardiac arrest from a presumed episode of pulmonary hypertension and required closed-chest cardiopulmonary resuscitation. Oliguric renal failure subsequently developed and necessitated 5 days of peritoneal dialysis. An acute rejection episode, suspected by atrial arrhythmias and supported by monocyte cell cycle analysis, was successfully treated on postoperative Day 12. The patient then steadily improved with complete resolution of the complications and was discharged on postoperative Day 50.

The fourth baby (HLHS) underwent uncomplicated OCT, but signs of cardiac tamponade developed 3 hours postoperatively. The sternum was sterilely opened at the bedside and a silicone rubber skin patch applied, which resulted in improved cardiac hemodynamics. Two days later, the myocardial swelling resolved with successful secondary sternotomy closure. The baby then had one successfully treated episode of rejection at postoperative Day 25 and was eventually discharged on postoperative Day 48.

The fifth baby (HLHS) had uncomplicated OCT and aortic arch reconstruction; however, the sternum could not be closed without cardiovascular compromise. A silicone rubber skin patch was placed in the operating room primarily. This resulted in a stable postoperative recovery, and secondary closure was completed 3 days later, after resolution of myocardial swelling. Subsequently, one episode of rejection was successfully treated on postoperative Day 15, and the patient was discharged on postoperative Day 43.

Because we chose not to perform percutaneous intramyocardial biopsies, evaluation of suspected rejection was based on clinical criteria that included unexplained fever, change in feeding habits, and alteration of activity level. Routine determinations of monocyte and lymphocyte replicative cell kinetics profiled cellular activity and served as a reliable index of clinical rejection. Electrocardiography and myocardial enzyme analysis were routinely performed, but were not helpful in determining early myocardial rejection. Echocardiography, however, was helpful in determining changes in fiber shortening when compared serially. We have no experience with gaited nuclear magnetic resonance imaging; however, easy access and early application of this diagnostic tool may help greatly in the early diagnosis of rejection by estimation of myocardial water content, accurate wall thickness measurement, and adenosine triphosphate analysis.

Pertinent donor–recipient comparisons are noted in Table 4. Body mass matchups varied by as much as 63%, but cardiac size silhouettes (by standard techniques) showed closer correlation. All had a negative lymphocytotoxic crossmatch, but only one had HLA compatibility.

The five surviving children are at home, doing well 30, 24, 19, 15, and 7 months after the operation, respectively. The hospital re-admission rate for infectious complications or rejection episodes was 0.91 admissions/patient/year and the rejection rate was 0.5 episodes/patient/year. The longest survivor has had three episodes of presumed clinical rejection (including the first one) and all these were successfully treated by steroid administration, without loss of function (by echocardiography) and with return of a quiescent cell cycle analysis. One infant received antilymphocytic monoclonal antibody therapy (OKT3) for clinical rejection that was associated with myocardial septal swelling and slight decrease in the echocardiographic fiber shortening measurement. These findings reversed and the child has survived 7 months postoperatively. Myocardial biopsies at the 1-year catheterization schedule showed no evidence of rejection in the three children in whom it was performed. Graft growth has been gradual and proportionate to the child's growth, and cardiac catheterization 1 year postoperatively showed normal cavitary pressure measurements without evidence of valvular dysfunction or anastomotic strictures (Figs. 7 and 8).

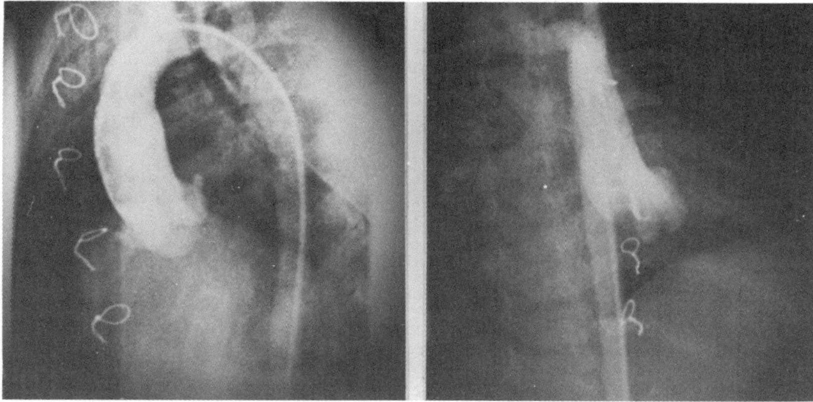

Figure 7: *Cineangiocardiograph oblique views showing postoperative aortic anatomy. The anastomotic site can be visualized, but no irregularities or stenosis are present. Reproduced with permission from Mavroudis et al.*[5]

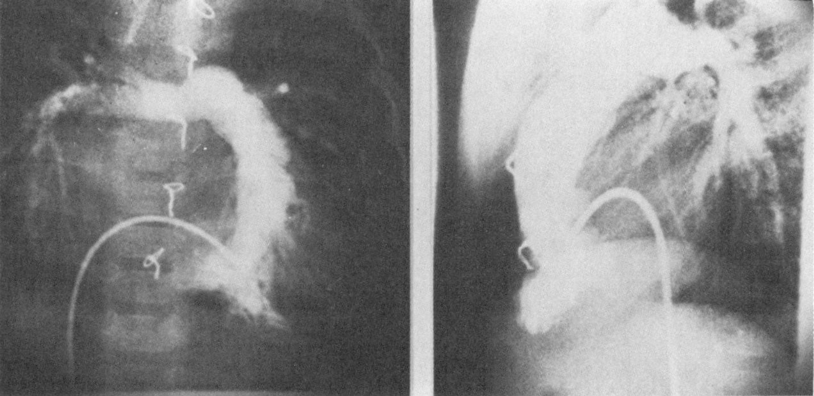

Figure 8: *Cineangiocardiograph oblique views showing postoperative pulmonary artery anatomy. The anastomotic site is not visualized and no stenosis or irregularities are present. Reproduced with permission from Mavroudis et al.*[5]

A New Classification

After reviewing our intraoperative results with infant OCT, it became obvious that extensive arch reconstruction in conjunction with OCT would be responsible for a higher incidence of intraoperative technical problems that could cause significant complications and death. Indeed, one of the deaths in this series was attributable to bleeding caused by the technical aspects of extensive arch reconstruction. In order to categorize these patients with HLHS, who may or may not require extended arch reconstruction with OCT, we retrospectively reviewed the charts and cineangiocardiograms of 38 patients with the spectrum of hypoplastic left heart syndrome from 1966 to 1986.[25] We defined the hypoplastic left heart syndrome as a spectrum of diseases that included those as described by Noonan and Nadas[26] and associates[27–32] as well as those with critical aortic stenosis and hypoplastic left ventricle.[27–29] All these patients had inadequate left ventricles[29] and depended, to various degrees, on the right ventricle and patent ductus arteriosus for pulmonary and systemic blood flow. Special consideration was paid to the size of the ascending aorta compared with the descending aorta and to the degree of coarctation of the aorta.

Two patterns of patients with hypoplastic left heart syndrome emerged, requiring different types of aortic reconstruction with OCT. Type I (32 patients) showed hypoplastic left heart, hypoplastic aortic arch, and coarctation. The coarctation in these patients was: discreet in 18 (Fig. 9), relative in 4 (Fig. 10), and indeterminate in 10. We originally made reference to these Type I patients in our clinical study,[5] where we subtyped them into Type IA for HLHS with discreet coarctation and Type IB for HLHS with relative coarctation. Because the distinction often can be arbitrary and because the same extensive arch reconstruction is necessary for both subtypes, we decided to omit subclasses within the Type I classification. Figure 11 represents Type II (6 patients) who showed: hypoplastic left heart, atretic (N = 1) or stenotic (N = 5), aortic valve, and adequately sized ascending aorta without coarctation. Adequately sized aorta was defined as a ratio of ascending aorta to descending aorta to be greater than 0.80. This ratio was chosen based on the measurements of two patients in our category of hypoplastic left heart syndrome (one with critical aortic stenosis and hypoplastic left heart; the other with aortic atresia, Fig. 12) and adequately sized aorta, who underwent successful orthotopic cardiac transplantation without arch reconstruction.[5] Cardiac catheterization in both patients, 1 year postoperatively, showed normal growth of the ascending aortic and transverse arch without evidence of ascending aortic stenosis by angiography or pressure measurements. Classification of the various forms of hypoplastic left heart syndrome has been

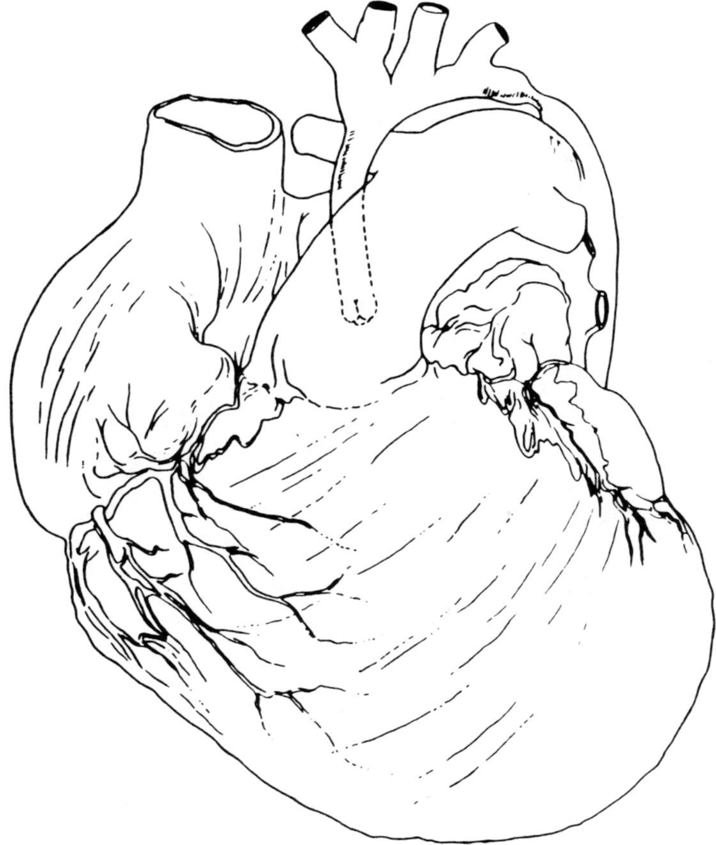

Figure 9: *Diagrammatic drawing showing Type I hypoplastic left heart syndrome characterized by hypoplastic left heart, hypoplastic aortic arch, and coarctation of the aorta. Reproduced with permission from Mavroudis et al.*[25]

based on patterns of hypoplasia of the ascending aorta, aortic valve, mitral valve, and left ventricle.[26–32] Although these classifications help the anatomists, embryologists, and pathologists to designate this spectrum of diseases, they do very little to help transplant surgeons relate the type of anomaly to the extent of operation necessary for eventual therapy and comparison of results.

We have described the surgical classification for the spectrum of hypoplastic left heart syndrome referable to OCT and aortic arch reconstruction. The originally described hypoplastic left heart syndrome

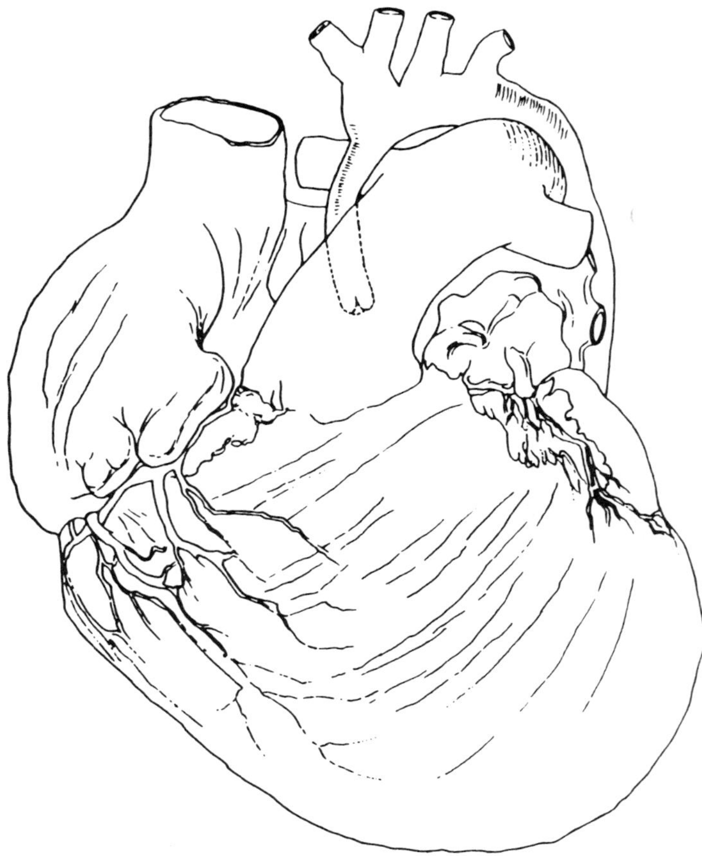

Figure 10: *Diagrammatic drawing showing Type I hypoplastic left heart syndrome characterized by hypoplastic left heart, hypoplastic aortic arch, and relative coarctation of the aorta. Reproduced with permission from Mavroudis et al.*[25]

introduced by Noonan and Nadas[26] has been expanded for our classification to include patients with severe aortic stenosis and hypoplastic left heart,[25] because this subgroup of patients represents a forma frusta of the original hypoplastic left heart syndrome with similar physiologic characteristics, natural history, and treatment options. The goal of this classification is to categorize these patients into a group that requires OCT only (Type II, Fig. 13) and a group that requires orthotopic cardiac transplantation and extensive aortic arch reconstruction

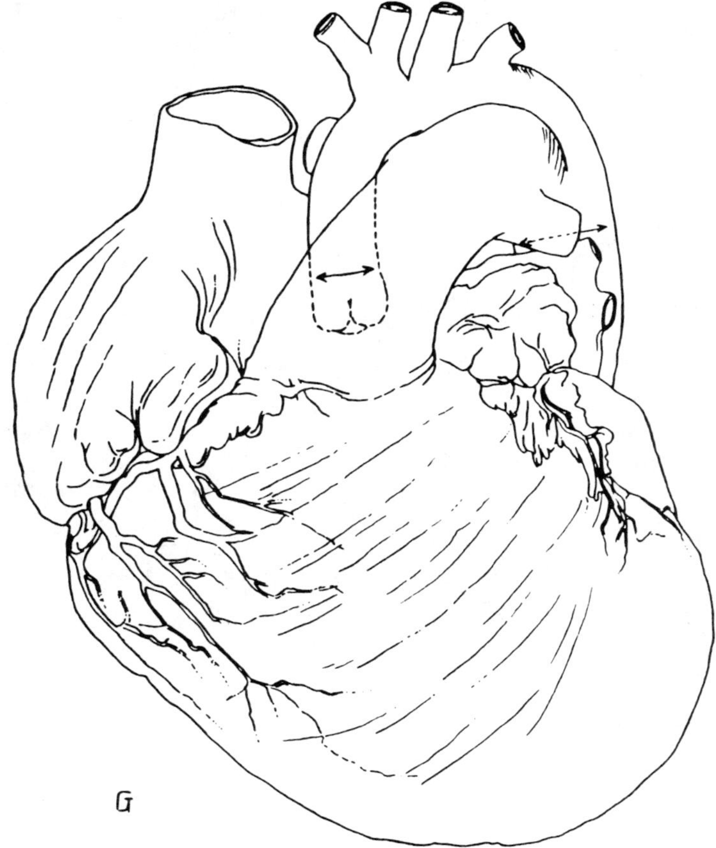

Figure 11: *Diagrammatic drawing showing Type II hypoplastic left heart syndrome characterized by hypoplastic left heart and adequately sized ascending aorta, which is defined by a ratio between the diameter of ascending aorta, just below the innominate takeoff (arrow), and the descending aorta, just downstream to the ductus arteriosus (arrow), of .80 or greater. The aortic valve may be fused (aortic atresia and hypoplastic left heart) or stenotic (critical aortic stenosis and hypoplastic left heart). Reproduced with permission from Mavroudis et al.*[25]

(Type I, Fig. 14). Surgeons can thus compare mortality and morbidity factors more accurately since OCT without aortic arch reconstruction would seemingly have fewer complications than OCT with aortic arch reconstruction.

The difference between discrete and relative coarctations is not

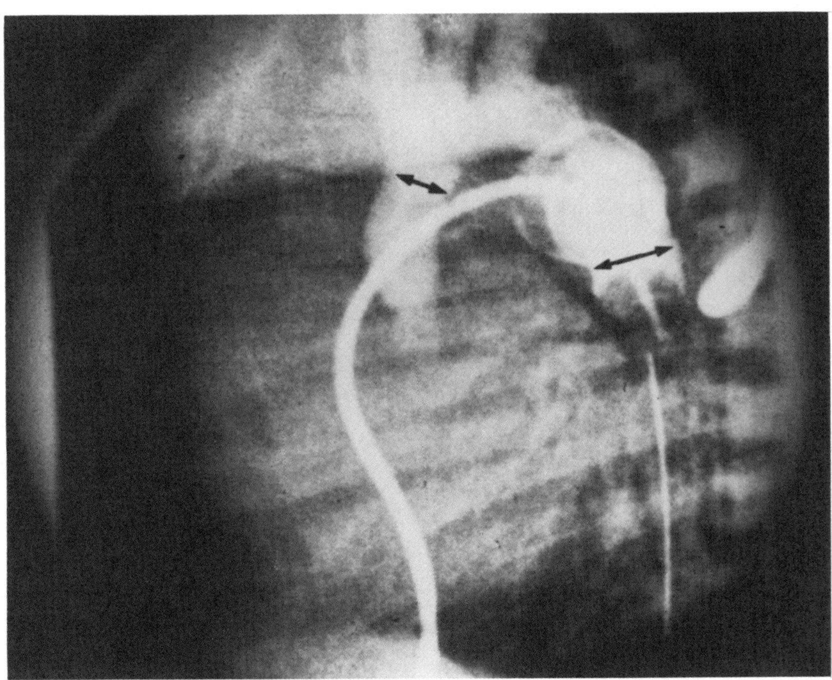

Figure 12: *Cineangiocardiogram showing Type II anatomy in a patient who underwent orthotopic cardiac transplantation without arch reconstruction. The aortic valve was fused (atresia), which was confirmed after explanation. The arrows refer to the measurements that were used to determine the adequately sized ascending aorta (see Figure 11). Reproduced with permission from Mavroudis et al.*[25]

critical since the same operation is required for both of these subtypes. In this retrospective analysis, 16 patients (42%) had discrete coarctations, 6 patients (16%) had relative coarctations, and in 10 patients (26%) distinction could not be made between the two. Similar findings related to the aortic arch and coarctation have been noted by other authors in postmortem studies.[31] We, therefore, recommend OCT with extended arch reconstruction at least 3–4 mm downstream of the ductus arteriosus to ensure adequate outflow in Type I patients.

The "adequately sized ascending aorta" requires clarification and definition. We have performed OCT without aortic arch reconstruction in two neonates with Type II hypoplastic left heart syndrome, who survived surgery and are achieving their normal growth and develop-

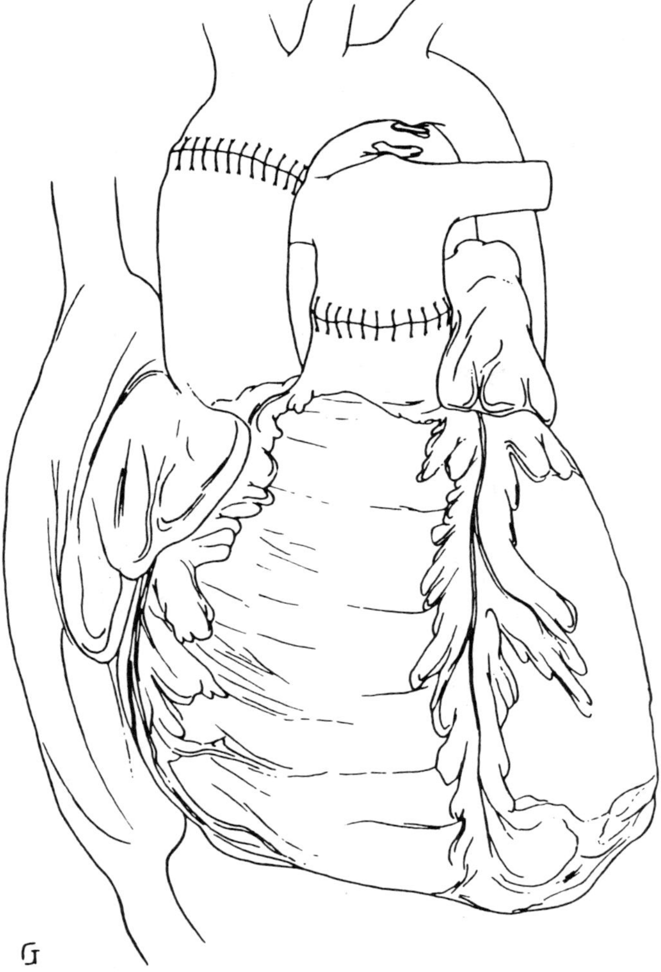

Figure 13: *Diagrammatic figure showing aortic anastomosis performed in conjunction with orthotopic cardiac transplantation for Type II patients. Reproduced with permission from Mavroudis et al.*[25]

mental milestones.[5] One of them had critical aortic stenosis, hypoplastic left ventricle without coarctation, and the other had aortic atresia, hypoplastic left ventricle without coarctation (Fig. 12). Our preoperative decision not to reconstruct the entire arch was a clinical one, in which we estimated that the outflow would be sufficient. In retro-

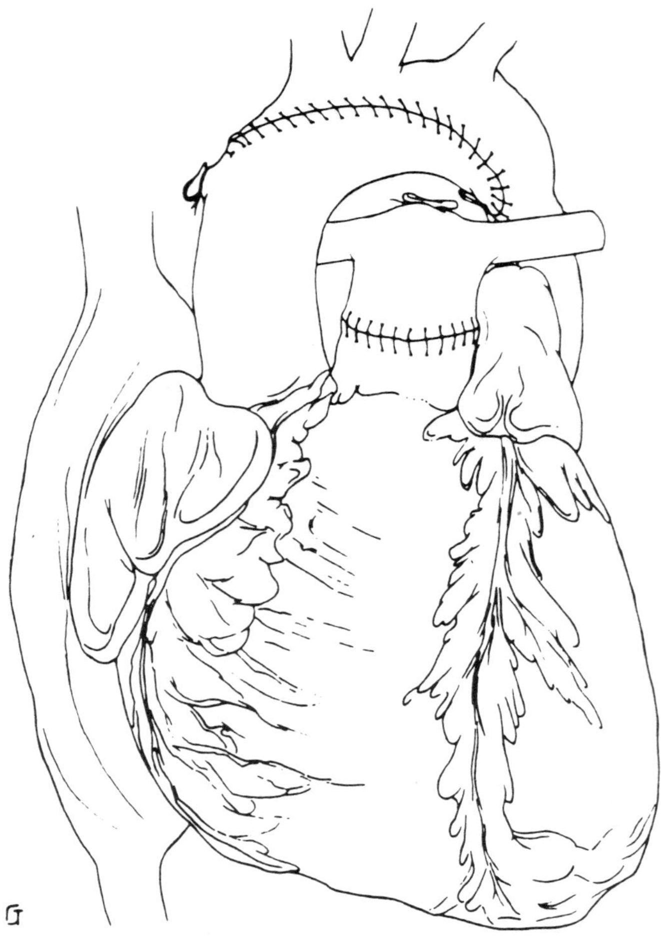

Figure 14: *Diagrammatic figure showing aortic arch reconstruction performed in conjunction with orthotopic cardiac transplantation for Type I patients. Reproduced with permission from Mavroudis et al.*[25]

spect, we measured the diameter of the ascending aorta just below the takeoff of the innominate artery and compared it with the diameter of the descending aorta, just distal to the ductus arteriosus, in the ratio: diameter of ascending aorta/diameter of descending aorta. We found the ratio was 0.83 in one patient and 0.81 in the other. We compared these findings to the six Type II patients in this retrospective analysis (Table 6) and found these patients had a ratio of 0.80 or better and

Table 6 Characteristics Of The Aortic Tract Complex*

	Aortic Valve Anatomy	Ratio†
Patient #1	Aortic atresia	.83
Patient #2	Severe aortic stenosis	.84
Patient #3	Severe aortic stenosis	.88
Patient #4	Severe aortic stenosis	.80
Patient #5	Severe aortic stenosis	.87
Patient #6	Severe aortic stenosis	.95

*Type II hypoplastic left heart syndrome patients defined as: hypoplastic left heart and adequately sized ascending aorta (AO/DO of .8 or greater); †Ratio: ascending aorta (AO) / descending aorta (DO), Reproduced with permission from Mavroudis et al.[25]

would probably have been suitable candidates for OCT without extensive arch reconstruction, based on our clinical findings.[5]

We already have experienced a Type I death due to technical problems with extended arch reconstruction, which most likely would not have occurred in a Type II patient. This new classification will allow surgeons to accurately compare mortality and morbidity figures as they relate to technical parts of the operation, which may, in the long term, help to improve the clinical results.

Discussion

Recent application of OCT to infants with severe forms of untreatable congenital heart disease has been shown to be effective in the short term.[2,5,6] The long-term uncertainty of survival and unpredictable complications, however, remain to be seen as these children grow and mature. As a result, we were careful to provide conscientious and informed consent for the families who were deciding on the proper course of action. This posture resulted in only half of the families desiring OCT for their babies. Although we thought the acceptance rate was low, we interpreted this as evidence of our espoused neutrality toward this method of therapy. The reasons for the refusals were multifactorial, surrounding complex outpatient care and philosophical objections based on whether this was the "right thing to do." Those families who accepted the transplant protocol were motivated and had extensive family support.

The most frustrating part of the transplant experience was the waiting period between the time the baby was listed on the organ procurement network and the time when a donor was available for transplantation. One only baby had severe complications from a 60-day wait, which resulted in severe neurologic deficit just before donor heart was available. This led to donor heart refusal because of the baby's hopeless condition. The rest of the babies (7 neonates, 1 infant) eventually received a donor heart (5 to 26 days) after organ procurement network listing. As this therapy becomes more acceptable and performed by more centers, the waiting period will obviously increase unless efforts are realized to increase the available donor pool. Besides donor availability, donor–recipient size compatibility will also represent a significant problem, because ideal donor–recipient size matches are not always available. Originally, we determined that a ± 30% body weight discrepancy would be acceptable for neonates; however, this considerably restricted our search for donors. We then examined the chest roentgenogram comparisons between donor and recipient and found that the cardiac silhouette sizes could better predict size compatibility than the actual body mass. This policy resulted in successful transplantation in three infants, despite larger donor-to-recipient size discrepancies of 63%, 50%, and 45%, respectively.

The operative approach to these infants is based on previously well-described principles.[3,17] The seven neonates underwent deep hypothermia and circulatory arrest with an average arrest time of 47 min for orthotopic cardiac transplantation. The one 11-month-old infant had bicaval cannulation with continuous moderate hypothermic perfusion. We found that removal of air from the heart was a significant problem and probably resulted in the death of our third patient, from coronary air embolism and myocardial swelling. Because of this, we instituted left ventricular, intracavitary cold saline instillation by placing a catheter through the left atrium into the left ventricle after the atrial anastomoses were completed.[33] In this manner, not only was myocardial preservation better served, but removal of air was also much more thorough. Since the introduction of this technique, we have had no difficulties with air embolism. Unlike previously reported cases,[2,6] our neonates with hypoplastic left heart syndrome required different degrees of aortic reconstruction. This operative experience prompted a 20-year review of our patients with hypoplastic left heart syndrome, which resulted in the new classification of hypoplastic left heart syndrome, referable to orthotopic cardiac transplantation and to the necessary extent of aortic arch reconstruction. As a result, two of our seven patients with hypoplastic left heart syndrome had large enough ascending aortas for a classic type of orthotopic cardiac transplantation, and the other five required extensive arch reconstruction as described by Bailey and his associates.[3]

We found that use of the silicone rubber skin patch[24] could provide a lifesaving maneuver when myocardial swelling occurs and the chest cannot be closed. We successfully used the silicone rubber skin patch in infants who had mild swelling of the myocardium. The skin patch was sutured tightly to the skin to prevent any leakage from the mediastinal structures. Two days later, after the myocardial swelling abated, it was removed and sternal closure was accomplished without difficulty. This maneuver can help stabilize the postoperative course in these patients when myocardial swelling or size discrepancy problems intervene.

Our immunosuppression treatment is based on acute and chronic triple-drug therapy, which is at variance with the chronic single-drug therapy proposed by Bailey and his associates.[2,6] Our reluctance to convert to a single-drug therapy has been based on our lack of HLA compatibility and our success with the present regimen. We, like Bailey and his associates,[2,6] believe that a decrease in the amount of steroids these patients receive is essential to long-term survival. As a result, we have been instituting every-other-day steroid therapy with decreasing doses in our older infants. The issue of acquired tolerance as a result of neonatal cardiac transplantation has not been settled. Clearly, these infants do not reject their hearts with the same immunologic competence that older children and adults do. The reasons for this are unknown at the present time and further research may determine the status of host tolerance in neonatal life. Whether these children will require less medication over a period of time to control rejection will also be of some interest for the future.

The diagnosis of rejection in the absence of myocardial biopsies was circumstantial in our series and based on clinical signs that were supported by determinations of monocyte cell cycle analysis and evaluation of the echocardiogram. Deviation from normal behavior, which included unexplained fever, change in feeding habits, and alteration of activity level, prompted a systematic search for active infection, nonevasive evaluation of cardiac function, and determination of monocyte cell cycle analysis. When infection was excluded and the cell cycle analysis showed increased cellular activity, the clinical signs were presumed to be due to rejection and the patient was treated with intravenous methylprednisolone. In one patient, the short methylprednisolone "pulse" (7.5 mg/kg) was not effective in reversing echocardiographic evidence of decreased ventricular function. This patient received intravenous OKT3 therapy with dramatic improvement in left ventricular function. This child went on to do quite well and is now 7 months postoperative without any signs of rejection in evidence by nonevasive means or by myocardial biopsy. The result of the infants responded to the methylprednisolone pulse and were presumed to have had a rejection episode. Although there is no one clinical or laboratory study specific for rejection, our approach has been to exclude the possibility of infection, while using clinical and laboratory evidence to arrive at the diagnosis. As technology has improved over this short period of time,[34–36] we have started to perform transcutaneous myocardial biopsies in these patients at 6 months of age. It is quite possible that, eventually, myocardial biopsies could be performed safely during the perioperative period.

Infant OCT for the severe forms of untreatable congenital heart disease has proved to be an effective and acceptable therapeutic procedure, even considering the unknown future, when compared with the natural history of the disease process for which OCT was applied. The short-term results have been encouraging in many centers. Clearly, more data must be accumulated to determine the long-term effects of immunosuppression.

Future Considerations

Recent advances in OCT have demonstrated the short-term success of this mode of therapy.[5,6] Future strides must be accomplished in the field of immunologic host control to avoid the concomitant complications of infection, coronary artery disease, and the threat of malignancy. The other, more acute, problem is donor availability, which has already caused pressure and competition for available hearts. Efforts to ease these problems have been attempted by Bailey and his associates,[1] who used baboon xenotransplantation and anencephalic homotransplantation.[6] The baboon transplantation experimentation failed due to erythrocyte incompatibility.[37] These, and other, unknown aspects of xenotransplantation must be explored before universal approval can take place. Xenotransplantation as a "bridge" to homotransplantation seems to be an attractive solution to the organ shortage problem, because the urgency of immediate transplantation can be served, to allow time for an eventual homotransplant. The obvious scientific problem with this approach centers around early control of rejection and host antibody induction caused by the xenograft, which may hinder eventual successful homograft transplantation. The economic, moral, and ethical dilemmas of this therapy are obvious and center around governmental and private financial reserves, objections from animal right's organizations, and knowing when to replace a well functioning xenograft with an unproven homograft.

The use of the anencephaly donor has also caused much controversy. Many view this as a partial solution to the inadequate donor pool,[38–40] whereas others object to their use of philosophical arguments and present brain-dead laws under which the anencephalics cannot be classified.[41] Although anencephalic organ donation is not practiced in the United States, Holzgreve and associates[42] of West Germany successfully transplanted kidneys from anencephalic donors without medical, political, or criminal incident. More recently, Bailey and associates performed an orthotopic cardiac transplant from an anencephalic donor from Canada.[43,44] In their case, however, they used life-support systems for the anencephalic infant and waited until standard "brain-dead" criteria were met.

In order to gather some data on this subject, we reviewed the clinical characteristics of all babies with anencephaly and hypoplastic left heart syndrome born in Kentucky from 1981 to 1985.[45] Forty-six neonates had HLHS (Fig. 15). Their average weight was 3.0 kg and all were anatomical and physiological candidates for OCT and aortic arch reconstruction, assuming donor availability and parental consent. In addition, there were 64 live births with anencephaly (Fig. 16). Thirty-three anencephalics weighed less than 2 kg, rendering them unlikely candidates for cardiac transplantation (Fig. 17). However, 31 weighed greater than 2 kg, making them reasonably sized candidates for neonatal organ transplantation. None of these anencephalic infants received any life-support measures after birth and lived for variable periods of time (Fig. 18). Forty-eight percent lived longer than 2 hours after birth, and all were dead within 2 weeks, confirming similar results published by Baird and Sadovnick.[46]

The data from this retrospective study show that enough anencephalic infants of appropriate size were born during the 5-year period to ease the demand for organ donors that were required from infants with hypoplastic left heart syndrome born during the same period.

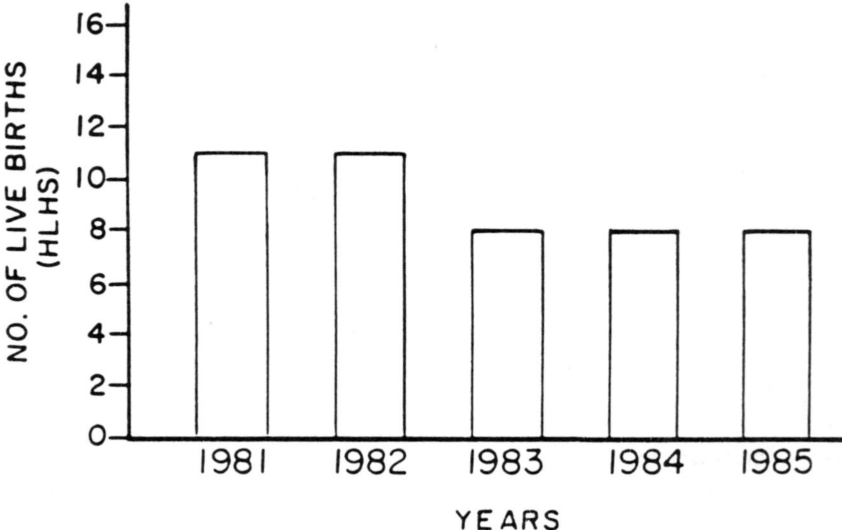

Figure 15: *Bar graph showing the number of patients per year diagnosed with hypoplastic left heart syndrome at Kosair Children's Hospital and University of Kentucky Chandler Medical Center from 1981–1985. HLHS = hypoplastic left heart syndrome. Reproduced with permission from Mavroudis et al.*[45]

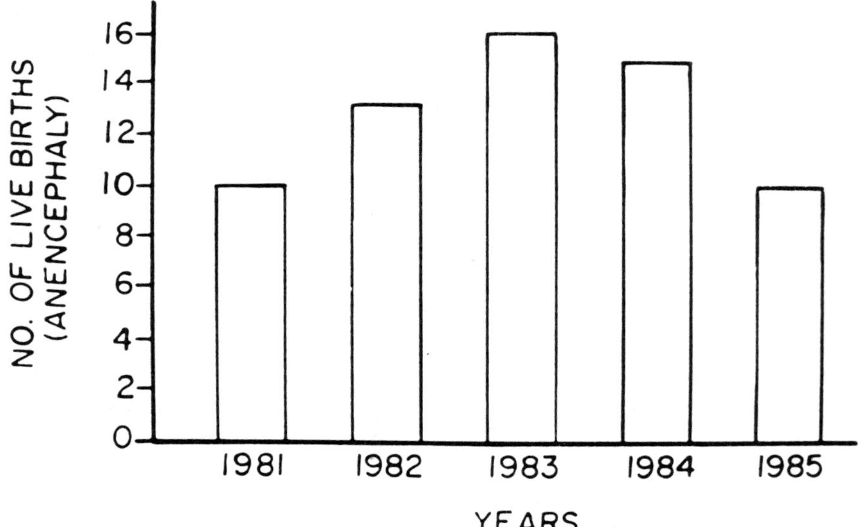

Figure 16: *Bar graph showing the number of patients per year diagnosed with anencephaly in Kentucky from 1981–1985. Reproduced with permission from Mavroudis et al.*[45]

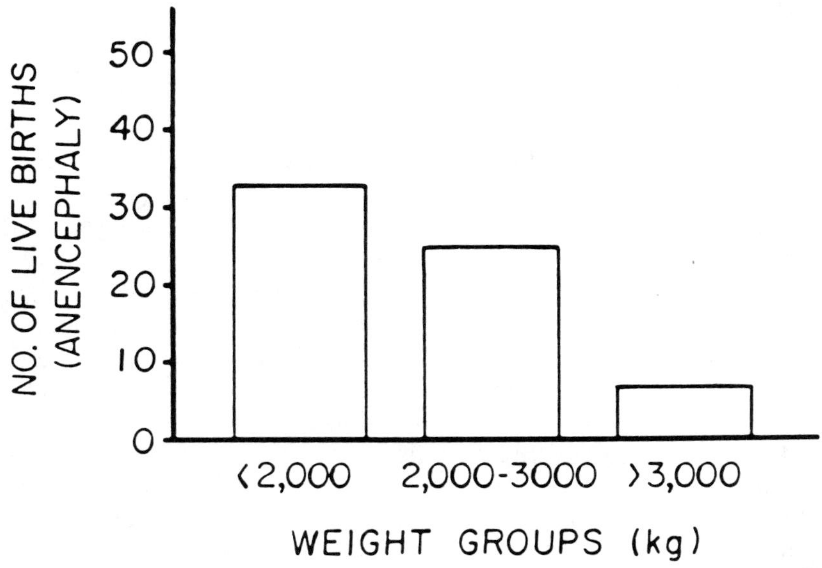

Figure 17: *Bar graph classifying anencephalics by weight groups (gm). Reproduced with permission from Mavroudis et al.*[45]

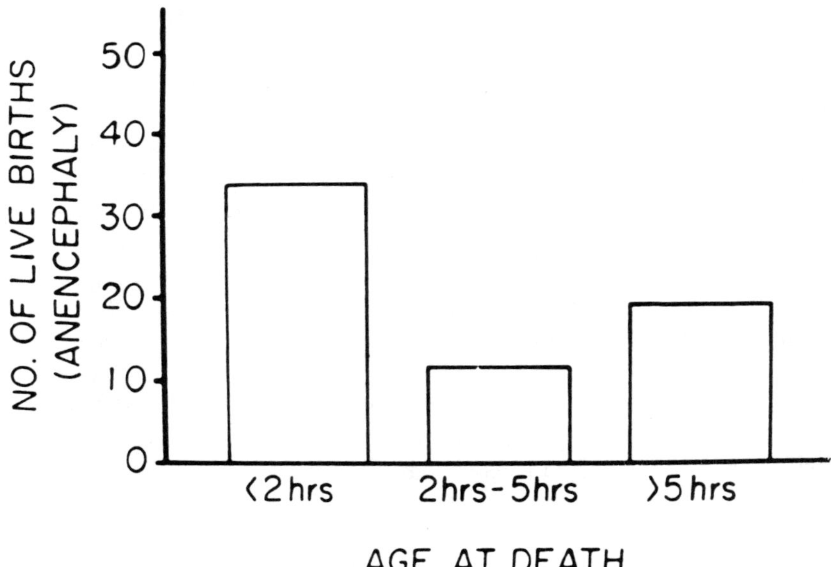

Figure 18: *Bar graph classifying anencephalics by age at death (hours). Reproduced with permission from Mavroudis et al.*[45]

Effective coupling of these groups could ameliorate the dilemma of organ shortage if applied nationwide to increase the pool and to allow for donor–recipient time, size, and blood type matchups.

The moral and ethical problems with this therapeutic approach, however, must be understood and debated. The protagonists who support anencephalic organ donations cite the moral duty of beneficence (to do good for others). They feel that a new brain-death category should be evolved or that a change in the uniform anatomical gift act should be enacted to allow organ transplantation of anencephalics, since they eventually die. They also feel that the donation should take place when the organs are at their physiologically optimal state. Moreover, the involved families are allowed some hope, since they see an opportunity to extend another life, thereby giving some purpose to an otherwise catastrophic and calamitous situation.

The antagonists cite three possible violations of the moral duty of nonmaleficence (do no harm). The first is derived from natural law tradition, which states that any offspring of a man and a woman, from the moment of conception, is human and, ipsofacto, a person. The anencephalic, therefore, is a non–brain-dead person and should not be used as organ donor.[41] Others, however, disagree and feel that the anencephalic is not a person because it cannot and never will interact with the environment.[47] The second possible violation of nonmaleficence is the issue of euthanasia (taking a life) before the potential donor is declared brain dead.[48] Acceptable medical practice has been to allow the anencephalic to die naturally. Whether euthanasia can be applied to anencephalics who undergo temporary life support for the purpose of organ transplantation is debatable and not entirely agreed upon. The third possible violation in nonmaleficence is expressed as the wedge or slippery-slope argument; that is, if an exception to the brain-dead law is made, will there be a moral drift in the direction toward using other neurologically impaired, non–brain-dead or nonanencephalic children for organ donation? The protagonists note that anencephaly is a unique neurologic case and can be defined in such a manner that would answer the slippery-slope argument.[38,39,47] Whatever the outcome of these scientific, moral, and ethical debates, it is quite clear that more dialogue must occur between physicians, ethicists, and legislatures to eventually solve these compelling problems.

References

1. Bailey LL, Nehlsen-Cannarella SL, Concepcion W, et al: Baboon-to-human cardiac xenotransplantation in a neonate. JAMA 1985, 254:3321.
2. Bailey LL, Nehlsen-Cannarella, Doroshow RW, et al: Cardiac allotransplantation in newborns as therapy for hypoplastic left heart syndrome. N Engl J Med 1986, 315:949.
3. Bailey L, Concepcion W, Shattuck H, et al: Method of heart transplantation for treatment of hypoplastic left heart syndrome. J Thorac Cardiovasc Surg 1986, 92:1.
4. Cooley DA, Frazier OH, Van Buren CT, et al: Cardiac transplantation in an 8-month-old female infant with subendocardial fibroelastosis. JAMA 1986, 256:1326.
5. Mavroudis C, Harrison H, Klein JB, et al: Infant orthotopic cardiac transplantation. J Thorac Cardiovasc Surg 1988, 96:912.
6. Bailey LL, Assaad AN, Trimm RF, et al: The Loma Linda University Infant Heart Transplant Group. Orthotopic transplantation during early infancy as therapy for incurable congenital heart disease. Ann Surg 1988, 208:279.
7. Bailey LL, Lacour-Gayet F, Perier P: Orthotopic cardiac transplantation in the neonate: Survival studies in a goat model. 1st ed. Proceedings of Beijing Symposium on Cardiothoracic Surgery. China Academic and John Wiley and Sons, Inc, New York 1982, pp. 342–350.
8. Bailey LL, Li ZJ, Lacour-Gayet F, et al: Orthotopic cardiac transplantation in the cyclosporine-treated neonate. Transplant Proc 1983, 15:2956.
9. Bailey LL, Li ZJ, Roost H, et al: Host maturation after orthotopic cardiac transplantation during neonatal life. Heart Transplant 1984, 3:265.
10. Bailey LL, Jang J, Johnson W, et al: Orthotopic cardiac xenografting in the newborn goat. J Thorac Cardiovasc Surg 1985, 89:242.
11. Turley K, Mavroudis C, Ebert PA: Cardiopulmonary bypass in the first week of life. Circulation 1982, 66(Suppl I):214.
12. Jamieson SW, Oyer P, Baldwin J, et al: Heart transplantation for end stage ischemic heart disease: The Stanford experience. Heart Transplant 1984, 3:224.
13. Griffith BP, Hardesty RL, Bahnson HT: Powerful but limited immunosuppression for cardiac transplantation with cyclosporin and low dose steroids. J Thorac Cardiovasc Surg 1984, 87:35.
14. Kaye MD, Ekombe SA, O'Fallon WM: The international heart transplantation registry: The 1984 report. Heart Transplant 1985, IV:290.
15. Norwood WI, Lang P, Castaneda AR, et al: Experience with operations for hypoplastic left heart syndrome. J Thorac Cardiovasc Surg 1981, 82:511.
16. Sade RM, Crawford FA Jr, Fyfe DA: Letters to the editor: Symposium on hypoplastic left heart syndrome. J Thorac Cardiovasc Surg 1986, 91:937.
17. Lower RR, Shumway NE: Studies on orthotopic homotransplantation of the canine heart. Surg Forum 1960, 11:18.
18. Galbraith RM, Galbraith GMP: Expressions of transferrin receptors on

mitogen-stimulated human peripheral lymphocytes: Relation to cellular activation and related metabolic events. Immunology 1981, 44:703.
19. Neckers LM, Cossman J: Transferrin receptor induction in mitogen-stimulated human T lymphocytes is required for DNA synthesis and cell division and is regulated by interleukin 2. Proc Natl Acad Sci USA 1983, 80:3494.
20. Suthanthiran M, Walle A, Darzynkiewicz Z, et al: Multiparameter analysis of cell activation in renal allograft recipients by flow cytofluormetry and by interleukin-2 production. Kidney Int 1984, 25:351.
21. Miller LW, Roodman ST, Tsai C, et al: Immune monitoring of interleukin 2 receptors (IL2R) in heart transplantation. J Heart Transplant 1986, 5:377.
22. Mohanakumar T, Hoshinaga K, Wood NL, et al: Enumeration of transferrin-receptor-expressing lymphocytes as a potential marker for rejection in human cardiac transplant recipients. Transplantation 1986, 42:691.
23. Braylan RC, Benson NA, Nourse V, et al: Correlated analysis of cellular DNA, membrane antigens and light scatter of human lymphoid cells. Cytometry 1982, 5:337.
24. Mavroudis C: Anatomical repair of transposition of the great arteries with intact ventricular septum in the neonate: Guidelines to avoid complications. Ann Thorac Surg 1987, 43:495.
25. Mavroudis C, Elbl E, Malias M, et al: Orthotopic cardiac transplantation in the neonate: Surgical classification for the spectrum of patients with hypoplastic left heart syndrome. Ann Thorac Surg (Submitted for publication).
26. Noonan JA, Nadas AS: The hypoplastic left heart syndrome: An analysis of 100 Cases. Pediatr Clin North Am 1985, 5:1029.
27. Bharrti S, Lev M: The surgical anatomy of hypoplastis of aortic tract complex. J Thorac Cardiovasc Surg 1984, 88:97.
28. Lev M: Pathologic anatomy and interrelationship of hypoplasia of the aortic tract complexes. Lab Invest 1952, 1:61.
29. Sinha SN, Rusnak SL, Sommers HM, et al: Hypoplastic left ventricle syndrome: analysis of thirty autopsy cases in infants with surgical considerations. Am J Cardiol 1968, 21:166.
30. Hawkins JA, Doty DB: Aortic atresia: Morphologic characteristics affecting survival and operative palliation. J Thorac Cardiovasc Surg 1984, 88: 620.
31. Roberts WC, Perry LW, Chandra RS, et al: Aortic valve atresia: A new classification based on necropsy study of 73 cases. Am J Cardiol 1976, 37:753.
32. Saied A, Folger GM Jr: Hypoplastic left heart syndrome. Am J Cardiol 1972, 29:190.
33. Baumgartner WA, Reitz BA, Oyer PE, et al: Cardiac homotransplantation. Curr Probl Surg 1979, 16:1.
34. Bhargava H, Donner RM, Sanchez G, et al: Endomyocardial biopsy after heart transplantation in children. J Heart Transplant 1987, 6:298.
35. Dunn JM, Cavarocchi NC, Balsara RK, et al: Pediatric heart transplanta-

tion at St. Christopher's Hospital for Children. J Heart Transplant 1987, 6:334.

36. Lurie PR: Editorial: Revision of pediatric endomyocardial biopsy technique. Am J Cardiol 1987, 60(4):368.
37. Bailey LL: Biologic versus bionic heart substitutes. Will xenotransplantation play a role? ASAIO Transactions 1987, 10:51.
38. Harrison MR: The anencephalic newborn as organ donor. Hastings Cent Rep 1986, April:21.
39. Harrison MR: Organ procurement for children: The anencephalic fetus as donor. Lancet 1986 Dec:1383.
40. Caplan AL: Should fetuses or infants be utilized as organ donors? Bioethics 1987, I:119.
41. Capron AM: Anencephalic donors: Separate the dead from the dying. Hastings Cent Rep 1987, Feb:5.
42. Holzgreve W, Beller FK, Buchholz B, et al: Kidney transplantation from anencephalic donors. N Engl J Med 1987, 316:1069.
43. Gianell DM: Anencephalic heart donor creates new ethics debate. Am Med News 1987, 3:47.
44. Annas GJ: From Canada with love: Anencephalic newborns as organ donors. Hastings Cen Rep 1987, XVII:36.
45. Mavroudis C, Willis RW, Malias M: Orthotopic cardiac transplantation for the neonate: The dilemma of the anencephalic donor. J Thorac Cardiovasc Surg 1989, 97:389–391.
46. Baird PA, Sadovnick AD: Survival in infants with anencephaly. Clin Pediatr 1984, 23:268.
47. Laberge JM: Letter to the Editor. Transplanting organs from anencephalic infants. Can Med Assoc J 1987, 137:473.
48. Arras JD, Shinnar S: Anencephalic newborns as organ donors: A critique. JAMA 1988, 259:2284.

Chapter 8

Immunosuppression Regimens for Pediatric Transplantation

Nicholas C. Cavarocchi and
Pierantonio Russo

History

The goals of any immunosuppression drug regimen includes prevention of allograft rejection, minimal drug side effects, avoidance of chronic medical complications and excellent long-term survival. Although there has been a dramatic increase in pediatric and adolescent transplantation in the United States and worldwide, an ideal immunosuppression regimen for children undergoing transplantation is still not available.

The development of pharmacologic immunosuppression has been through numerous stages pre- and postintroduction of cyclosporine. In the precyclosporine era, drugs used clinically differed from cyclosporine in that they were nonspecific and indiscriminately cytotoxic against all dividing cells, including immunocompetent cells. Azathioprine, first used in 1961[1,2] in combination with corticosteroids, formed the earliest immunosuppressive regimens.[3] In 1966, antilymphocyte globulin (ALG) was introduced as a third and short-term immunosuppressive adjunct.[4,5] Other protocols developed to include substitution of azathioprine with cyclophosphamide and the use of total lymphoid irradiation (TLI).[4–7] Although ALG and TLI basically eliminate only immunocompetent cells, they are nonspecific within that cell group.

The cyclosporine era has ushered in a more advanced era of immunoregulation as the first compound to be active against a specific

From *Heart Transplantation in Children,* edited by Jeffrey M. Dunn, M.D. and Richard M. Donner, M.D. © 1990, Futura Publishing Company, Inc., Mount Kisco, NY.

subgroup of immunocompetent cells.[8,9] This specificity of action distinguishes cyclosporine from azathioprine and corticosteroids, which suppress all immunocompetent cells. Cyclosporine was initially used alone in 1978–1979; corticosteroids were added in 1980 in combination with cyclosporine. In the early 1980s, cyclosporine and corticosteroids were the standard immunosuppression regimen for most cardiac recipients worldwide, no matter what age.

In 1985, the early results of the randomized protocol[10] of cyclosporine and corticosteroids versus cyclosporine and azathioprine demonstrated no significant differences between protocols. At the same time, there was growing dissatisfaction with the chronic side effects, such as nephrotoxicity and hypertension, which developed in patients on high-dose cyclosporine and corticosteroids. In 1985–1986, we saw the birth of the triple immunosuppression regimen of low-dose cyclosporine, corticosteroids, and azathioprine, which remains the standard of choice for the majority of adult cardiac recipients. Continuing concern over the acute and chronic side effects of maintenance corticosteroids in children, combined with the encouraging results from the Papworth group[10] led to the development of a regimen of cyclosporine and azathioprine. Cyclosporine and azathioprine is presently the accepted regimen of choice for infants and adolescents.

Diagnosis of Rejection

Orthotopic heart transplantation in infants, children, and young adults is an increasingly successful alternative to conventional medical and surgical palliative therapy.[11–13] However, the unique concept of recipient size, growth and development, and susceptibility to infection have raised questions about traditional methods for diagnosing and treating acute and chronic rejection in children. In the adult patient, clinical evaluations[14] and noninvasive laboratory procedures[14,15] have been useful for suggesting the presence of acute graft rejection; however, endomyocardial biopsy remains the standard by which therapeutic decisions are made.[14,16,17] Alternate approaches to endomyocardial biopsy for identifying the presence of acute graft rejection have received much attention in the adult and pediatric transplant literature. Specifically, clinical signs of illness,[13,14] abnormalities of electrocardiography,[14] and echocardiography, as well as radionuclide studies,[15] have been used as substitutes to biopsy. It is generally agreed that the sensitivity and specificity of these methods must approach 100% because failure to identify acute rejection or to exclude infection and other causes for illness may result in graft loss and patient death. This is of particular importance in the pediatric population where nonspecific clinical signs of illness may be difficult to interpret. Natural exposure and immunization to control pathogens may not have been acquired, whereas immaturity of the immune system may aggravate the response to immunosuppressive therapy resulting in a greater incidence of serious infection.

Our experience with endomyocardial biopsies supports the current feeling that clinical symptoms, abnormalities on physical examination, increasing cardiomegaly, and diminished pump performance on echocardiography do not fulfill the desired criteria for sensitivity and specificity. Further, repeated endomyocardial biopsies performed via the femoral vessels in infants and children can be performed safely, efficiently, and with a minimum of discomfort.[18–20]

Endomyocardial biopsies are scheduled and performed, irrespective of clinical status, according to the following protocol: weekly for the first month, biweekly for the next 2 months, and monthly for the following 6 months. Additional biopsies were performed when the clinical course or noninvasive testing were suggestive of acute graft rejection and again 1 week following treatment of the rejection episode. Factors that led to nonscheduled biopsies were fever, fatigue, the presence of a gallop rhythm, tachycardia, arrhythmias, edema on physical examination, increasing cardiomegaly on chest x-rays, or diminished pump performance on echocardiography. In several infants, tachypnea, fussiness, or poor feeding were additional criteria for performing nonscheduled biopsies. Clinical signs and symptoms, either alone or in combination, led to the diagnosis of acute allograft rejection, proven by endomyocardial biopsy, in approximately 50% of recipients. It is important to remember that all new signs and symptoms are rejection until proven otherwise and endomyocardial biopsy should be performed to rule out the diagnosis. The diagnosis of rejection on endomyocardial biopsy was defined as per Billingham.[21]

Noninvasive testing such as electrocardiography and radionuclide studies has not supplanted endomyocardial biopsy as the procedure of choice for evaluating acute rejection in infants and children. Therefore, we firmly believe that the most predictable method of detecting rejection remains the endomyocardial biopsy, no matter what the age of the recipient.

Treatment of Rejection

Effective treatment of rejection episodes is the mainstay of prolonging graft and patient survival after cardiac transplantation. The overall incidence of rejection is reported to range between 0.23 to 3.42 episodes per patient by various institutions.[22–24] Episodes of rejection are routinely diagnosed by endomyocardial biopsy,[21] with moderate or severe acute rejection episodes being treated by a variety of modalities that can include pulsed intravenous or oral corticosteroids, increased cyclosporine dosage, antithymocyte globulin (ATGAM), OKT3 (Ortho Diagnostic Systems, Raritan, N.J., U.S.A.), or combinations of the above.

The administration of either intravenous or oral corticosteroids is our treatment of choice for a patient with moderate or severe acute myocardial rejection without hemodynamic compromise. It has been demonstrated by Michler et al.[25] and others[26] that moderate acute rejection can be effectively treated with oral corticosteroids and does not require large dose of intravenous corticosteroids. Over time, we have evolved three corticosteroid treatment protocols for moderate acute rejection (Table 1). All moderate rejection episodes ≤30 days after transplantation and all severe rejection episodes regardless of time after transplantation were treated with the intravenous Solu-Medrol protocol. Any severe rejection episodes with hemodynamic compromise were treated with a combination of intravenous Solu-Medrol and horse antithymocyte globulin. All moderate acute rejection episodes >30 days postoperatively were treated with one of three proto-

Table 1 Protocol for Rejection Episodes

Rejection	Cyclosporine	Azathioprine	Prednisone	HATG
Early	NC	NC	Protocol 1	3–5 day (10 mg/kg/day) I.V. if resistant or severe rejection)
Late	NC	NC	Protocol 1 Protocol 2 Protocol 3	

Early ≤ 30 days, late >30 days; NC = no change; HATG = horse antithymocyte globulin; I.V. = intravenous; Protocol 1 = Solu-Medrol (I.V.) 15 mg/kg/day × 3 days; Protocol 2 = oral prednisone (1 mg/kg/day) weaned over 3 weeks to 0.2 mg/kg/day as maintenance or stopped; Protocol 3 = oral prednisone (1.5 mg/kg/day) × 5 days and stopped.

Table 2 Cost of Rejection Therapy

Solu-Medrol (intravenous)—hospitalized	$2800.00
Solu-Medrol (intravenous)—at home	$ 500.00 to $1,000.00
Prednisone (oral) (3-week taper)	$ 3.00
Prednisone (oral) (5 days)	$ 2.00

cols: I.V. Solu-Medrol; 3-week taper of oral prednisone; or a 5-day course of oral prednisone (Table 1).

Analysis of our treatment for moderate rejection in our combined adult and pediatric population demonstrated an equal success in all three protocols (approximately 75% in all three). There was a significant increase in side effects (glucose intolerance, mood swings, weight gain, hypertension) in the intravenous corticosteroid group versus both oral corticosteroid therapy protocols. No patient in our pediatric series developed any significant infection during rejection therapy with any of the protocols. The cost for intravenous versus oral corticosteroid therapy is also significantly different (Table 2). Solu-Medrol given at home or by in-patient nursing services was still significantly more expensive than oral corticosteroids.

We have not found it necessary to use monoclonal antibodies or other forms of immunosuppressive therapy to treat acute rejection episodes in any of our pediatric population. A number of our patients who were on the cyclosporine and azathioprine protocol did require conversion to triple-drug immunosuppression for a short period of time to clear up a resistant rejection episode. The majority of patients have been weaned back off the oral corticosteroid and remain only on double therapy, that is, cyclosporine and azathioprine.

Chemical Immunosuppression

A series of elegant innovative experiments performed by Billingham and his colleagues[27] demonstrated that graft rejection is in the immune process. Furthermore, these workers found it was possible to manipulate the developing immune system so that it would accept foreign organs. Although donor-specific immunosuppression is the goal for those seeking to control allograft rejection, the clinician faced with the urgency of treating fatal disease, often in the young, has turned to the less subtle approach of nonspecific immunosuppression. When one considers the amount of time, effort, and money invested in trying to control the immune system, the number of active agents discovered is depressingly small. The pharmacologic agents that have been shown to be of clinical value in organ transplantation are azathioprine, corticosteroids, and cyclosporine A. Antithymocyte globulin and antilymphocyte globulin will not be discussed.

Azathioprine

In 1961, azathioprine, one of the agents closely related to 6-mercaptopurine, was found to have superior therapeutic index for immunosuppression in dogs with renal allografts.[28] The results were variable, but long-term survivors were reported. Azathioprine was first used in clinical organ transplantation by Murray and his colleagues[29] in 1963 and has since proven to be one of the most valuable immunosuppressive drugs in recipients of organ allografts. Although it is capable of acting as an antimetabolite for the biologic roles of both adenine and hypoxanthine, details of the important pharmacologic actions of azathioprine as an immunosuppressive are not known. The side effects can be serious, particularly depression of the bone marrow and all its cellular elements. Some patients may develop megaloblastic anemia when treated with azathioprine. The drug can be hepatotoxic in man. There is still considerable variation in the clinical use of azathioprine concerning optimal dosage, but in general most patients are given the maximal dose they can tolerate without evidence of toxic marrow suppression. Most patients will tolerate 2–3 mg/kg/day orally.

Corticosteroids

Various researchers have found that cortisol diminished the inflammatory response[30] and also increased long-term survival in animals with renal allografts[31] Murray et al.[29] combined azathioprine with corticosteroids in a program of renal transplantation that for the first time, showed a reasonable expectation of survival in recipients of kidneys from cadaver donors. This combination of azathioprine and corticosteroids became the anchor of immunosuppression from 1961 until the introduction of cyclosporine in 1978. Although the exact mechanisms of the actions of corticosteroids as an immunosuppressive agent are unknown, it is thought to be an anti-inflammatory drug that leads to the sequesterization of lymphocytes and monocytes into the lymphatic tissue. It has also been shown to block the production of interleukin-1 and interleukin-2. As with both azathioprine and corticosteroids, there is lack of agreement as to the best way of using the medications. For many years, very high doses of corticosteroids were routinely given, but the excellent results obtained with relatively low doses of corticosteroids by McGowan al.[32] in Belfast has led many clinicians to reappraise this policy. Presently, the minimal amounts of corticosteroids are used for maintenance, and increased doses are used to treat rejection episodes. A great deal of debate has evolved concerning the usage of long-term corticosteroids in infants and children and its effects on growth and development, physical appearance, and chronic medical complications. Children maintained on chronic corticosteroids for any indication will have the side effects of long-term therapy. Therefore, the transplant community has attempted to maintain its pediatric populations on cyclosporine and azathioprine only. Although corticosteroids are added for rejection episodes, it has been relatively easy to maintain children on cyclosporine and azathioprine without using high doses of either medication. In general, children off corticosteroids do not show signs of chronic corticosteroid usage and have demonstrated and maintained normal growth curves. As with any disease process, a major illness or increase in immunosuppression may result in a fall in the growth curve for that individual.

There are a number of possible side effects to corticosteroids. These include Cushing's syndrome, induction of diabetes mellitus, ulcer disease, bone necrosis, cataracts, weight gain, acne, and hypertension. In general, it has been a policy to reduce corticosteroids to the minimum dose required to avoid rejection episodes. Discontinuing corticosteroids completely from a patient who has been on chronic immunosuppression may result in an acute rejection episode.

Although many promising new agents have been developed in the laboratory and some of them have been given to patients with organ grafts, none have had the therapeutic impact of the combination of azathioprine and corticosteroids. It must be remembered that although the mechanisms of corticosteroid action as an immunosuppressive agent are unknown, it works well to prevent rejection.

Cyclosporine

A major contributing factor to the significant progress in the field of transplantation has been the introduction of cyclosporine into clinical practice. Both U.S. and worldwide experience of those transplant centers that have been using cyclosporine as a long-term antisuppressive therapy suggest that cyclosporine is now the immunosuppressive agent of choice in solid-organ transplantation. Study results from these centers revealed that cyclosporine therapy is associated with superior patient and graft survival in liver and heart transplant recipients[33–35] and with improved graft survival in renal allograft recipients,[36–40] compared to results achieved with traditional immunosuppressive agents. This dramatic improvement in survival has been realized without an increase in mortality and morbidity.

Other benefits attributed to the use of cyclosporine include a reduction in both the frequency and severity of rejection,[37,39,41] a reduction in the overall incidence of infection,[39,42] and a reduction in the incidence of life-threatening infection.[33,37,38,42,43] The use of cyclosporine may also allow for reduction in steroid usage, which has been reported to result in excellent survival rates without corticosteroid-related side effects.[44,45] This reduction in corticosteroid dosage may be particularly beneficial in children. In one study in which cyclosporine was used in combination with low-dose corticosteroids, significantly improved graft survival was achieved and normal growth rate was reported in 28 children receiving renal allografts who were followed for more than 1 year posttransplant.[46] These factors, together with the improved survival rates seen in patients treated with cyclosporine, contributed to a significantly higher rate of patient rehabilitation, fewer hospital readmissions, and reduced cost.[36,41,47] Perhaps the most important advantage to consider is the improved quality of life that will be achieved in transplant patients treated with cyclosporine.

Unlike the traditional immunosuppressive agents, the mechanism of action by which cyclosporine interferes and interrupts the rejection process is highly specific. Current data suggest that cyclosporine exerts its effect by selectively and reversibly inhibiting the interleukin-2 driven proliferation of activated T lymphocytes.[48–50] Specifically, cyclosporine impairs interleukin-2 production and thereby suppresses proliferation and generation of cytotoxic lymphocytes, while sparing T suppressor cell subpopulations.[48,49] The persistence of suppressor cells in vivo suggests that these cells are critical to promotion of allograft tolerance.[48] In immunosuppressive doses, cyclosporine is not myelosuppressive.[48] There are a number of drug interactions that can occur with cyclosporine. There are drugs that may decrease cyclosporine concentration, such as phenytoin, phenobarbital, rifampin, isoniazid, and intravenous trimethoprim and sulfadimidine. There are also a number of drugs that may increase cyclosporine concentration, such as ketoconazole, erythromycin, Dantrazole, and high-dose methylprednisolone. There are also a number of potential drug interactions to cyclosporine that may affect renal functions. Cyclosporine should be used cautiously in patients taking other drugs that may affect renal function, particularly in patients taking aminoglycosides, amphotericin B, and trimethoprim, alone or in combination with sulfamethoxazole.

Cyclosporine can be clearly distinguished from other immunosuppresants because its action is specific and selective, and its effects are reversible. Compared with traditional therapy, treatment with cyclosporine results in superior or improved patient and graft survival rates in renal, liver, and heart transplant patients. In patients generally considered at high risk, such as the elderly, diabetic, retransplants, and poorly managed patients, the use of cyclosporine has resulted in excellent survival rates. Additional advantages of cyclosporine over traditional therapy include greatly reduced mortality from rejection; fewer late-occurring rejection episodes; fewer chronic irreversible rejection episodes; and fewer severe infections. Adverse reactions, such as nephrotoxicity, are dose dependent and reversible with dosing reduction. Patient management can be facilitated with individual dosages based on serum creatinine and drug levels. The corticosteroid-sparing effect of cyclosporine helps with steroid-related side effects, such as growth impairment in children and cushingoid symptoms. Finally, cyclosporine has resulted in shorter hospital stays and fewer readmissions, resulting in significant cost reduction to the transplant patient.

Immunosuppression Protocols at St. Christopher's Hospital for Children

Cardiac transplantation was first performed at St. Christopher's Hospital for Children in 1985. At that time, the immunosuppression protocol consisted of maintenance cyclosporine and corticosteroids for all patients. In 1986, the maintenance immunosuppression protocol at our institution was changed to two basic protocols divided by age. The immunosuppression protocol for children $\geq$14 years of age was exactly similar to our adult protocol (Table 3). A second immunosuppression

Table 3 Immunosuppression Protocol for Children ≥14 Years

	Cyclosporine	Prednisone	Azathioprine	ATG
Initial	2–5 mg/kg P.O.	1 mg/kg off CC	1.5 mg/kg/day P.O./I.V.	HATG × 5 days I.V. (10 mg/kg/day)
Maintenance	Increase according to creatinine, CYA level.	1 mg/kg/day in 2 divided doses, taper to 0.2 mg/kg/day over 4 weeks	1.5–2.0 mg/kg/day P.O., adjusted to WBC	

P.O. = oral; I.V. = intravenous; CC = cross clamp; HATG = horse antithymocyte.

protocol was developed for all children ≤14 years of age (Table 4). Both protocols used similar initial induction therapy. In the initial therapy, patients received 2.0 to 5.0 mg/kg of cyclosporine by mouth 1 hour prior to surgery. If the patient had evidence of renal insufficiency, no cyclosporine was used at all for the first 48 hours. Azathioprine was consistently given to all patients prior to the transplant procedure. Corticosteroids were also consistently used on all patients for the first 24 hours. Antithymocyte globulin was also given to all patients postoperatively. Horse antithymocyte globulin is administered intravenously over 4–6 hours via a central line.

Maintenance therapy in the immunosuppression protocols differed significantly in the fact that oral corticosteroids were not part of chronic immunosuppression for those children under the age of 14. In the protocol for the children less than 14 years of age, cyclosporine and azathioprine were not increased in relationship to the protocol used for

Table 4 Immunosuppression Protocol for Children ≤14 Years

	Cyclosporine	Prednisone	Azathioprine	ATG
Initial	2–5 mg/kg P.O.	10 mg/kg off CC	1.5 mg/kg/day P.O./I.V.	HATG × 5 days I.V. (T cells ≤1%) (10 mg/kg/day)
Maintenance	Increase according to creatinine CYA level.	10 mg/kg I.V. q8h × 3 then discontinue	1.5–2.0 mg/kg/day P.O., adjusted to WBC	

P.O. = oral; I.V. = intravenous; CC = cross clamp; HATG = horse antithymocyte.

the children greater than age 14. In the initial experience of Yacoub, 90% of his recipients who were maintained on cyclosporine and azathioprine were maintained off steroid at 1 year. At 4 years, this number had decreased to approximately 75%. Hypertension and nephrotoxicity, however, continued to be a problem in his experience and our own.

No matter which protocol the patient is maintained on, it is our policy to attempt to maintain the lowest dose of immunosuppression possible, while still preventing rejection episodes. All patients' immunosuppressions are reviewed after endomyocardial biopsy, and whichever drug is causing them the most side effects is weaned to its lowest possible dose. We attempt to maintain all patients on low-dose cyclosporine to prevent many of its short- and long-term side effects. If the patient is on prednisone, we attempt to get the prednisone down to 0.1 to 0.2 mg/kg/day. At the same time, azathioprine is maintained fairly constantly at 1.5 to 2.0 mg/kg/day if the patient's white blood cell count and platelets are maintained. In general, azathioprine rarely needs to be adjusted because patients find an equilibrium with the drug and their white cell count response. Despite high doses of azathioprine, patients can develop a white blood cell count or fever with most bacterial and/or viral infections. At the present time, we do not have any pediatric patients who have been weaned entirely off cyclosporine because of renal problems. However, our adult experience is such that some patients have been weaned off cyclosporine and are maintained on conventional immunosuppression of corticosteroids and azathioprine. How low one is able to take any of the immunosuppressive drugs without causing a rejection episode is really unknown. In general, when we are actively decreasing immunosuppressive drugs, we may in fact increase the frequency of surveillance biopsies so we can keep a close track of whether or not an asymptomatic rejection episode is occurring.

Although we have gone through numerous assay techniques for cyclosporine, we are not very satisfied with any of the present techniques. Cyclosporine levels do not correlate with rejection episodes in cardiac transplant recipients. Early in our experience, when we relied more heavily on cyclosporine levels, we were impressed by the difficulty in maintaining adequately serum or blood cyclosporine levels with traditional cyclosporine dosage. Our younger patients frequently required two to three times the adult dose. This would appear to be secondary to a more rapid cyclosporine metabolism, the high doses resulting in excessively high peaks soon after an oral dose and excessively low troughs 10–12 hours later. This can be effectively countered by changing the dosage regimen in children to every 8 hours rather than the traditional every 12 hours. By doing so, an adequate trough cyclosporine level—used by us and others to monitor cyclosporine dosage—can be maintained with a lower total cyclosporine dosage/day and decreased side effects, such as renal dysfunction and cyclosporine-induced seizures that seem to be associated in certain children with the "peak" level. As we have come to rely less on cyclosporine levels, but manage cyclosporine dosage based on level of injection, renal function (serum creatinine and creatinine clearance), and hypertension, we have relied less on t.i.d. dosage than in the past. Therefore, we do not find it imperative to maintain a standard cyclosporine level in all our patients. We do not find that cyclosporine levels correlate well with renal function, and therefore, we pay particular attention to the serum creatinine and adjust cyclosporine dosage according to creatinine and results of biopsy.

References

1. Murray JE, Merrill JP, Dammin GJ, et al: Kidney transplantation in modified recipients. Ann Surg 1962, 156:337.
2. Murray JE, Merrill JP, Harrison JH, et al: Prolonged survival of human-kidney homografts by immunosuppressive drug therapy. N Engl J Med 1963, 268:1315.
3. Starzl TE, Marchioro TL, Waddell WR: The reversal of rejection in human renal homografts with subsequent development of homograft tolerance. Surg Gynecol Obstet 1963, 117:385.
4. Starzl TE, Iwatsuki S, Shaw BW Jr, et al: Factors in the development of liver transplantation. Transplant Proc 1985, l7(Suppl II):107.
5. Starzl TE, Porter KA, Iwasaki Y, et al: The use of heterologous antilymphocyte globulin in human renal homotransplantation. In Wolstenholme GEW, O'Connor M, eds: Antilymphocytic Serum. J & A Churchill Ltd, London, 1967, pp. 4-34.
6. Starzl TE, Putnam CW, Halgrimson CG, et al: Cyclosphamide and whole organ transplantation in human beings. Surg Gynecol Obstet 1971, 133: 981.
7. Najarian JS, Ferguson RM, Sutherland DER, et al: Fractionated total lymphoid irradiation as preparative immunosuppression in high risk renal transplantation. Ann Surg 1982, 196:442.
8. Hess AD, Tutschka PJ, Santos GW: The effect of cyclosporin A on T-lymphocyte subpopulations. In White DJG, ed: Cyclosporin A: Proceedings of an International Conference on Cyclosporin A. Elsevier Biomedical Press, Amsterdam, 1982, pp. 209-231.

9. Cohen DJ, Loertscher R, Rubin MF, et al: Cyclosporine: A new immunosuppressive agent for organ transplantation. Ann Intern Med 1984, 101:667.
10. Cavarocchi NC, Hakin M, Cory-Pearce R, et al: A prospective randomized trial of cyclosporine and low-dose prednisolone vs. cyclosporine and azathioprine. Presented at Sixth Annual Scientific Session of the International Society of Heart Transplantation, New York, April 26, 1985.
11. Pennington DG, Sarafian J, Swartz M: Heart transplantation in children. J Heart Transplant 1985, 4:441.
12. Fricker FJ, Griffith BP, Hardesty RL, et al: Experience with heart transplantation in children. Pediatrics 1987, 79:138.
13. Bailey LL, Nehlsen-Cannarella SL, Doroshaw RW, et al: Cardiac allotransplantation in newborns as therapy for hypoplastic left heart syndrome. N Engl J Med 1986, 315:949.
14. Caves PK, Stinson EB, Billingham ME, et al: Serial transvenous biopsy of the transplanted human heart. Improved management of acute rejection episodes. Lancet 1974, 1:821.
15. Hess ML, Hastillo A, Wolfgang TC, et al: The noninvasive diagnosis of acute and chronic cardiac allograft rejection. J Heart Transplant 1982, 1:31.
16. Billingham ME: Diagnosis of cardiac rejection by endomyocardial biopsy. J Heart Transplant 1982, 1:25.
17. Pomerance A, Stovin P: Heart transplant pathology: The British experience. J Clin Pathol 1985, 38:146.
18. Lurie PR, Fujita M, Neustein HB: Transvascular endomyocardial biopsy in infants and small children: Description of a new technique. Am J Cardiol 1978, 42:453.
19. Anderson JL, Marshall MW, Allison SB: The femoral venous approach to endomyocardial biopsy: Comparison with internal jugular and transarterial approaches. Am J Cardiol 1984, 53:833.
20. Bhargara H, Donner RM, Sanchez G, et al: Endomyocardial biopsy after heart transplantation in children. J Heart Transplant 1987, 6:298.
21. Billingham M: Diagnosis of cardiac rejection by endomyocardial biopsy. Heart Transplant 1:25.
22. Halbrook H, Bechman S, Hormuth D, et al: Heart transplant at a private institution: A two year experience. Heart Transplantation 1985, 4:353.
23. Reemsta K, Hardy M, Drusin R, et al: Cardiac transplantation changing patterns in evaluation and treatment. Ann Surg 1985, 202:418.
24. Caves PK, Stinson E, Billingham M, et al: Percutaneous transvenous endomyocardial biopsy in human heart recipients. Experience with a new technique. Ann Thorac Surg 1973, 16:324.
25. Michler R, Smith C, Drusin R, et al: Reversal of cardiac transplant rejection without massive immunosuppression. Circulation 1986, 74(Suppl III):III-68.
26. Renlund D, O'Connell J, Gilbert E, et al: Feasibility of discontinuation of corticosteroid maintenance therapy in heart transplantation. J Heart Transplant 1987, 6:71.

27. Billingham RE, Brent L, Medawar PB: The antigenic stimulus in transplantation immunity. Nature 1956, 178:514.
28. Calne RY, Murray JE: Inhibition of the rejection of renal homografts in dogs with Burroughs-Wellcome. Surg Forum 1961, 12:118.
29. Murray JE, Merill JP, Harrison JH, et al: Prolonged survival of human kidney homografts by immunosuppressive drug therapy. N Engl J Med 1963, 268:1315.
30. Dempster WJ: Kidney homotransplantation. Br J Surg 1953, 40:447.
31. Zukoski CF, Callaway JM, Rhea WG: Prolonged acceptance of a canine renal allograft achieved with prednisolone. Transplantation 1965, 3:380.
32. McGowan MG, Douglas JF, Brown MD, et al: Advantages of low dose steroid from the day after transplantation. Transplantation 1980, 29:287.
33. Macoviak JA, Oyer PE, Stinson EB, et al: Four-year experience with cyclosporine for heart and heart-lung transplantation. Transplant Proc 1985, l7(Suppl II)97.
34. Griffith BP, Hardesty RL, Trento A, et al: Five years of heart transplantation in Pittsburgh. Heart Transplantation 1985, 4:489.
35. Starzl TE, Iwatsuki S, Shaw BW Jr, et al: Orthotopic liver transplantation in 1984. Transplant Proc 1985, 17:250.
36. Milford EL, Kirkman RL, Tilney NL, et al: Clinical experience with cyclosporine and azathioprine at Brigham and Women's Hospital. Am J Kidney Dis 1985, 5:313.
37. Feduska NJ, Melzer J, Amend WJC, et al: Clinical management of immunosuppressive therapy for cyclosporine-treated recipients of cadaver kidney transplants at one to six months. Transplant Proc 1986, 18(Suppl I):136.
38. The Canadian Multicentre Transplant Study Group: A randomized clinical trial of cyclosporine in cadaveric renal transplantation: Analysis at three years. N Engl J Med 1986, 314:1219.
39. Canafax DM, Simmons RL, Sutherland DER, et al: Early and late effects of two immunosuppressive drug protocols on recipients of renal allografts: Results of the Minnesota randomized trial comparing cyclosporine versus antilymphocyte globulin azathioprine. Transplant Proc 1986, 18(Suppl I):192.
40. Johnson RWG: Cyclosporine in cadaveric renal transplantation: Three-year follow-up of a European multicentre trial. Transplant Proc 1986, 18:1229.
41. Kahan BD, Kerman RH, Wideman CA, et al: Impact of cyclosporine on renal transplant practice at the University of Texas Medical School at Houston. Am J Kidney Dis 1985, 5:288.
42. Ferguson RM, Sommer BG: Cyclosporine in renal transplantation. A single institutional experience. Am J Kidney Dis 1985, 5:296.
43. Johnson RWG, Wise MH, Bakran A, et al: A four-year prospective study of cyclosporine in cadaver renal transplantation. Transplant Proc 1985, 17: 1197.
44. Calner RY, White DJG, Evans DB, et al: Cyclosporin A in cadaveric organ transplantation. Br Med J 1981, 282:934.

45. Calne RY, Rolles K, White DJG, et al: Cyclosporin A initially as the only immunosuppressant in 34 recipients of cadaveric organs. Thirty-two kidneys, two pancreases, and two livers. Lancet 1979, ii:1033.
46. Brodehl J, Offner G, Hoyer PF, et al: Cyclosporin A in pediatric kidney transplantation and its effect on posttransplantation growth. Nephron 1986, 44:26.
47. Rettig RA, Barker C: Costs and benefits of cyclosporine therapy in renal transplantation. Am J Kidney Dis 1985, 5:344.
48. Cohen DJ, Loertscher R, Rubin MF, et al: Cyclosporine: A new immunosuppressive agent for organ transplantation. Ann Intern Med 1984, 101:667.
49. Wish JB: Immunologic effects of cyclosporine. Transplant Proc 1986, 18(Suppl II):15.
50. Buurman WA, Ruers TJM, Daemen IAJJM, et al: Cyclosporin A inhibits IL 2-driven proliferation of human alloactivated T cells. J Immunol 1986, 136:4035.

Chapter 9

Cyclosporine Metabolism and Pharmacokinetics in the Pediatric Heart Transplant Patient

Leslie M. Shaw, Carolyn Viewig, Leona Fields, and Jeffrey M. Dunn

Introduction

In studies of the pharmacokinetics of cyclosporine (CsA), it has been shown that there is appreciable variation in the absorption and elimination rates of the drug.[1–5] Investigations such as these and others were usually done within the first 2 weeks after transplant surgery while the patient was still hospitalized. Thus, it is possible that the other significant changes in the patient's hemodynamic, liver, renal, and gastrointestinal functions might account for at least some of the interpatient variation in CsA absorption and elimination. In the described study, we evaluated the oral pharmacokinetics and metabolism of CsA in five pediatric patients with stable hemodynamic, liver, renal, and liver function 10 weeks to 2.5 years after heart transplant surgery.

Methods

The patients included in this study were adolescent heart transplants ranging from 15 to 20 years of age. All the patients were free of infections and had stable cardiac, renal, liver, and gastrointestinal

From *Heart Transplantation in Children*, edited by Jeffrey M. Dunn, M.D. and Richard M. Donner, M.D.

function at the time of the study. Each patient fasted for at least 8 hours before receiving an oral dose of CsA. The first meal was consumed between 2 and 3 hours after drug administration. The age, sex, drug dosage, transplant date, pharmacokinetic study date, and time of drug administration are summarized in Tables 1 and 2. Blood specimens were drawn into EDTA vacutainer tubes at the following times in relation to the CsA dose: 1 hour before and 1, 2, 3, 4, 6, 8, 10, 12, 16, and 23 hours after for Patients 1 to 4. In the case of Patient 5, an additional tube of blood was collected at 20 hours after drug administration.

The blood specimens were stored at 4°C if they were to be analyzed within 5 days or at −20°C when stored for greater lengths of time prior to assay. On the day of assay, the specimens were well mixed at room temperature. A 1-mL aliquot of each blood specimen was subjected to ether extraction as described by Kahn et al.[6] The final dried extract was dissolved in 0.35 mL of the HPLC mobile phase. HPLC analysis of the extract was performed essentially according to the method described by Rosano et al.[7] Chromatographic separation of CsA and metabolites 17, 1, 21, and 8 was achieved using a DuPont cyanopropyl column (250 × 4.6 mm) maintained at 65°C and a mobile phase consisting of acetonitrile/water/methanol (38/59/3) at a flow rate of 1.5 mL/min.

Parent CsA was measured in aliquots of the well-mixed blood specimens by the Sandimmune monoclonal-specific radioimmunoassay.[8] We used the principle of reverse superposition to generate single-dose curves from the observed blood concentrations.[9] The area under the CsA concentration versus time curve (AUC), the first moment of the AUC (AUMC), mean residence time (MRT), the elimination rate constant (Kel), and elimination half-life for each patient was determined using the model-independent LAGRAN pharmacokinetics program.[10] The elimination rate constants and elimination half-lives were determined in LAGRAN pharmacokinetics program by linear

Table 1. Patient Data

Patient	Age	Sex	Transplant Date	Study Date	Time of CsA Dose
1	15	F	03/12/85	03/12/85	1235
2	20	M	10/16/86	09/10/87	1640
3	19	M	04/02/86	09/16/87	0800
4	18	M	05/15/86	09/21/87	1250
5	15	M	07/19/87	09/28/87	0800

Table 2. Cyclosporine Pharmacokinetic Data

Patient	Weight (kg)	CsA Dose (mg/kg)	C_{min}* (mg/L)	C_{max} (mg/kg)	T_{max} (hr)	Kel (hr^{-1})	AUC (mg/L)·hr	MRT** (hr)	$T^1/2$ (hr)	AUC*** (Norm)	Comments
1	46	7.0	247	631	4	0.059	8906	19.3	11.7	27.8	Smooth rise to peak starting at 1 hour postdose.
2	110	8.5	168	1310	4	0.061	5956	12.9	11.3	6.3	Essentially no absorption for 3 hours postdose, followed by a rapid rise to the peak concentration.
3	70	6.9	252	513	6	0.057	3019	16.2	12.2	6.3	Essentially no absorption for 3 hours postdose, followed by a rapid rise to the peak concentration.
4	72	5.8	148	852	6	0.086	8777	12.4	8.1	20.9	Smooth rise to the peak starting at 1 hour postdose.
5	59	7.5	579	2156	2	0.053	12880	13.7	13.0	29.3	Rapid rise to the peak concentration at 2 hours postdose.

*The concentration of cyclosporine in blood 1 hour before the stated oral dose was administered; **Mean residence time; ***Area under the CsA concentration versus time curve normalized to 1 mg of the CsA dose.

least squares analysis of the CsA concentrations obtained in the terminal phase including the 12-hour through the 23-hour samples. The MRT, which is the average time that CsA molecules reside in the body, was determined from the relationship,

$$MRT = \frac{AUMC}{AUC}.$$

Results

As noted in Table 2, there was significant variation in the apparent absorption of CsA. For Patients 1, 4, and 5, blood concentrations began to rise above the predose values at 1 hour after drug administration. However, for Patient 5, the initial rise in CsA concentration was rapid, peaking at 2 hours, whereas for Patients 1 and 4, the initial rise was more gradual, with peak concentrations at 4 and 6 hours, respectively. On the other hand, a considerable lag time was observed in Patients 2 and 3. CsA concentrations increased only slightly (from a predose value of 168 μg/L to a value of 184 μg/L at 3 hours postdose) or decreased slightly (from 252 μg/L to 211 μg/L at 3 hours postdose), respectively, and then rapidly increased to peak values of 1,310 μg/L and 513 μg/L at 4 and 6 hours postdose, respectively. The time from drug administration to the time at which maximal concentrations were attained ranged from 2 to 6 hours for the five patients. Maximal concentrations (C_{max}) ranged from 513 to 2,156 μg/L. Elimination half-lives ranged from 8.1 to 13.0 hours and mean residence times (MRT) ranged from 12.4 to 19.3 hours.

Figure 1 illustrates the log concentration versus time profiles for CsA, M17, M1, and M8 obtained for Patient 2 over the 24-hour pharmacokinetic study period (see Table 3 for trough blood concentrations of cyclosporine CsA and metabolites and estimated elimination half-lives determined in each of the five patients). When compared to the CsA and M1 curves, that of M17 is much flatter. For this patient, the maximal M17 concentration of 513 μg/L, attained 6 hours after drug administration, was only 1.9 times the 23-hour trough value of 268 μg/L.

The relative concentrations of M17 and CsA changed significantly throughout the dose interval with the maximal M17/CsA value of 2.0 occurring at 23 hours and the lowest M17/CsA value of 0.37 occurring

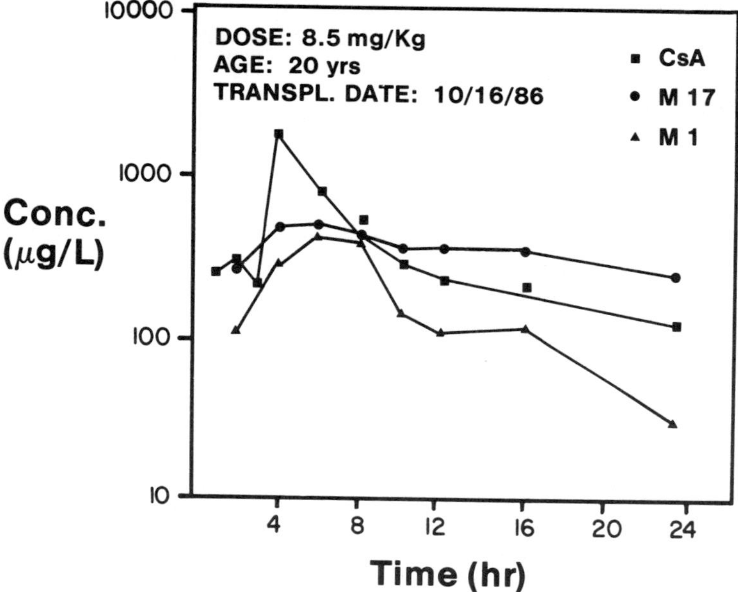

Figure 1: *Semilog plot of concentration versus time for Patient 2. The concentrations of CsA, M17, M1, and M9 were measured in the patient's blood by the procedures described in text.*

Table 3. Cyclosporine Metabolite Concentrations and Elimination Half-Lives

	Trough* Blood Concentrations					Elimination Half-Lives		
Patient	CsA	M17	M1	M21	M8	CsA**	M17***	M1***
1	205	96	66	72	14	11.7	10.2	6.3
2	133	268	30	N.D.***	34	11.3	27.7	6.0
3	107	348	51	N.D.	44	12.2	9.3	4.3
4	114	297	37	N.D.	46	8.1	22.1	6.8
5	307	319	68	N.D.	N.D.	13.0	16.5	7.7
$\bar{X}$	173	266	50		34	11.3	17.2	6.2
±SD	±84	±99	±17		±15	±1.9	±7.8	±1.2

*Concentrations in blood samples obtained 23 hours after the CsA dose; **Determined from the slope of the linear least squares line fitted to the log CsA concentration vs. time values from 12 through 23 hours after the oral dose of CsA was given; ***Determined from the slope of the linear least squares line fitted to the log (M17 or M1) concentration vs. time values from 10 through 23 hours after the oral dose of CsA was given; N.D. = none detected.

4 hours after CsA administration. Similar behavior was observed for Patients 3, 4 and 5.

In contrast, CsA concentrations in Patient 1 were higher than the corresponding values for M17 for all time points throughout the dose interval. The maximal M17/CsA value of 0.72 for this patient was achieved 16 hours after drug administration and the lowest value was 0.36 at 1 hour after drug administration. In this patient, the maximal M17 concentration of 393 μg/L, attained 4 hours after drug administration, was 3.6 times higher than the 23-hour trough value of 96 μg/L. Thus, not only were this patient's M17 values lower than CsA concentrations, but there were much greater changes in this metabolite's concentration throughout the dose interval (Fig. 1).

Discussion

Oral-dose pharmacokinetics of CsA was evaluated in five heart transplant recipients with stable cardiac function. Of the pharmacokinetic parameters investigated, the least variable was the elimination half-life. The values obtained for Patients 1 to 5 were 11.7, 11.3, 12.3, 8.1, and 13.0 hours, respectively. On the other hand, the maximal CsA concentrations varied extensively in relationship to the corresponding predose value (C_{max}/C_{min}): 2.6, 7.8, 5.8, 2.0, and 3.7, respectively. Furthermore, the time to reach maximal concentration (T_{max}) varied from 2 to 6 hours after drug administration: 4, 4, 6, 6, 2 hours for Patients 1 to 5, respectively. In our five patients, the extensive variation in the ratio C_{max}/C_{min} and in T_{max}, coupled with the much lower degree of variation of the rate of elimination, suggests that absorption of the drug is highly variable. Considerable variation in absorption and in terminal half-life has been observed in several studies of different groups of transplant patients.[1–5] However, since these studies were performed in hospitalized patients within the first 2 weeks after surgery, some of the observed variation could have been the result of their changing physiologic status. The results for these five patients indicate that even in clinically stable heart transplant patients there is considerable interpatient variation in apparent absorption of cyclosporine.

The metabolites that appeared in the blood of these patients in the greatest concentration were M17 and M1. At twenty-three hours, postdose concentrations of M17 were significantly higher than concentrations of M1. Furthermore, the mean 23-hour trough concentration of M17 (266 μg/mL) was 1.5 times the corresponding mean CsA concentration value of 173 μg/mL. In a study of cyclosporine metabolism in 24 renal transplant patients, the mean 12-hour trough M17 concentration was 1.7 times the mean CsA concentration.[11] Thus, the prominence of M17 appears to be a consistent finding, at least in heart and kidney transplant patients. In liver transplant patients, in fact, predose M17 concentrations in blood of up to 5.4 times the corresponding CsA concentrations have been observed.[12]

The pharmacologic and clinical significance of CsA metabolites is currently controversial. Several investigators have shown that metabolite 17 and several other metabolites have either very low or no immunosuppressive activity in several in vitro tests of immunosuppression.[13–15] On the other hand, Freed and co-workers have shown that M17 has significant immunosuppressive activity in comparison to CsA in several in vitro test systems.[16] The reason for the discrepant results is not apparent but could be the result of the use of different lymphocyte cell populations with differing sensitivities to CsA. In an in vivo rat model, the oral CsA dose required to produce a 50% inhibition of the antibody response against sheep erythrocytes was 3 mg/kg/day, whereas 50 mg/kg/day of orally administered M17 was ineffective.[14] A limitation in the latter study was the observed fivefold lower bioavailability of M17 in comparison to CsA,[14] making direct dose–response comparisons impossible.

With respect to the toxicity of CsA metabolites, only a few studies have been reported and this is another controversial subject. In a rat model, equivalent doses of M17 and CsA were administered by three routes (oral, subcutaneously, or intraperitoneally) for 4 weeks. Based on serum creatinine and BUN determinations and histological evaluation, there was no evidence for production of renal toxicity produced by M17, whereas CsA produced significant changes in the biochemical and histologic measurements of nephrotoxicity.[14] A limitation of this study is the lack of specific measurement of M17 in comparison to CsA in the rats' blood during the course of the study. In an in vitro test system, M17 had no effect on the growth of cultured renal tubule cells, whereas CsA produced a significant depression of their growth.[17] Further studies of the pharmacologic activity and clinical significance of M17 and other CsA metabolites will be required in order to determine their immunosuppressive activity and toxicity in man.

Editors Note

The efficacy of cyclosporine has made cardiac transplantation a more reasonable clinical modality and has thus afforded the opportunity for pediatric transplantation. Cyclosporine is not without its complications, including renal dysfunction, systemic hypertension, CNS seizures, and cardiac fibrosis. Each of these complications described in the adult population has been experienced in our pediatric population. If we are to succeed with pediatric transplantation, these complications must be controlled not for a few years as in the adult population but for decades.

In addition, we and others have observed significant differences in the pharmacokinetics of our pediatric heart transplantation patients compared to our older patients. Without a good understanding of the pharmacokinetics, it can indeed be impossible to maintain adequate cyclosporine levels without significant side effects.

References

1. Ptachcinski RJ, Venkataramanan R, Rosenthal JT, et al: Cyclosporine kinetics in renal transplantation. Clin Pharmacol Ther 1985, 38:296.
2. Ptachcinski RJ, Burckart GJ, Rosenthal JT, et al: Cyclosporine pharmacokinetics in children following cadaveric renal transplantation. Transplant Proc 1985, 18:766.
3. Yee GC, Lennon TP, Gmur DJ, et al: Age-dependent cyclosporine: Pharmacokinetics in marrow transplant patients. Clin Pharmacol Ther 1986, 40:438.
4. Burckart GJ, Starzl T, Williams L, et al: Cyclosporine monitoring and pharmacokinetics in pediatric liver transplant patients. Transplant Proc 1985, 17:1172.
5. Shaw LM, Bowers L, Demers L, et al: Critical issues in cyclosporine monitoring: Report of the task force on cyclosporine monitoring. Clin Chem 1987, 33:1269.
6. Kahn GC, Shaw LM, Kane MD: Routine monitoring of cyclosporine in whole blood and kidney tissue using high performance liquid chromatography. J Anal Toxicol 1986, 10:28.
7. Rosano TG, Freed BM, Cerilli J, et al: Immunosuppressive metabolites of cyclosporine in the blood of renal allograft recipients. Transplantation 1986, 42:262.
8. Sandimmune package insert. Sandoz Ltd, Balse Switzerland
9. Bauer LA, Gibaldi M: Computation of model-independent pharmacokinetic parameters during multiple dosing. J Pharm Sci 1983, 8:978.

10. Rocci ML, Jusko WJ: LAGRAN program for area and moments in pharmacokinetic analysis. Comp Prog Biomed 1983, 16:203.
11. Rosano TG, Free BM, Pell MA, et al: Cyclosporine metabolites in human blood and renal tissue. Transplant Proc 1986, 18(Suppl V):35.
12. Shaw, LM: Unpublished observation.
13. Maurer G: Metabolism of cyclosporine. Transplant Proc 1985, 17(Suppl I):19.
14. Ryffel B, Hiestand P, Foxwell B, et al: Nephrotoxic and immunosuppressive potentials of cyclosporine metabolites in rats. Transplant Proc 1986, 18(Suppl V):41.
15. Schlitt HJ, Christians U, Wonigeit K, et al: Immunosuppressive activity of cyclosporine metabolites in vitro. Transplant Proc 1987, 19:4248.
16. Freed BM, Rosano TG, Lempert N: In vitro immunosuppressive properties of cyclosporine metabolites. Transplantation 1987, 43:123.
17. Cole E, Skorecki K, Cheung F, et al: Cyclosporine in contrast to a cyclosporine metabolite specifically inhibits growth of renal cells in culture. Transplant Proc 1988, 20(Suppl III):732.

Chapter 10

Steroids and Growth in Children

Angelo M. DiGeorge

Corticosteroids, because of their immunosuppressive properties, are frequently administered to patients who have had organ transplants. Although most of the details of the mechanism of this action remain to be elucidated, it is clear that these agents are lympholytic, resulting in decreased size of thymus, spleen, and lymph nodes. The T lymphocytes are the major target cells; corticosteroids block the egress of these cells out of the bone marrow, resulting in decreased delayed hypersensitivity responses. In addition, this class of steroids has potent anti-inflammatory effects. They inhibit the primary antibody response, inhibit activation of macrophages, and interfere with production of various inflammatory mediators such as prostaglandins and leukotrienes.

Effect on Growth

The doses of corticosteroids required to obtain desired levels of immunosuppression are greater than their physiologic endogenous production and, therefore, induce undesirable effects.[1] Corticosteroid excess is catabolic, thereby inducing negative nitrogen balance with resultant loss of tissue mass. If administration of pharmacologic doses

From *Heart Transplantation in Children,* edited by Jeffrey M. Dunn, M.D. and Richard M. Donner, M.D.

is prolonged, they also cause osteopenia by inhibiting calcium absorption from the gastrointestinal tract as well as by decreasing osteoblastic activity. The sum of these effects results in inhibition of normal growth in children. Even before corticosteroids became clinically available as therapeutic agents, it was known that a major manifestation of Cushing's syndrome in children is impaired growth and short stature.[2] The cause for this syndrome is the excessive endogenous production of cortisol due to adrenal cortical tumors or adrenal hyperplasia secondary to excessive secretion of ACTH. Removal of the cortisol excess in affected children results in the resumption of normal growth.

Do Corticosteroids Affect Growth Hormone?

Current knowledge of the endocrine control of growth is incomplete despite recent advances. Because pituitary growth hormone is one of the major factors promoting normal growth, plasma levels of growth hormone have been measured in children with corticosteroid-induced growth retardation. However, a variety of such studies have established that secretion of growth hormone is normal, thus eliminating suppression of growth hormone as a mechanism for the growth failure associated with corticosteroid excess. This conclusion is further supported by studies in which administration of growth hormone to children with corticosteroid-induced growth failure did not promote normal growth. These observations suggested the possibility of a state of peripheral resistance to growth hormone under these conditions and led to the investigation of somatomedin generation. The action of growth hormone is mediated by the stimulation of a group of peptides known as somatomedins, the most important of which are IGF-I (insulin-like growth factor) and IGF-II. These peptides promote protein and collagen synthesis and are the principal mediators by which growth hormone enhances growth. Serum levels of IGF in 49 patients with Cushing's disease, including 13 children, were in the normal range for controls of the same age.[3] Normal IGF levels also have been found in patients during treatment with corticosteroids. Thus, IGF deficiency cannot account for the growth failure associated with corticosteroids. Although levels of somatomedin are normal, when levels of their bioactivity are measured, there is a significant decrease as soon as 6 hours after a dose of steroid and a return to the predose level by 24 hours.[4] This effect appears to be directly related to an increase in somatomedin inhibitory activity. Current evidence suggests that corticosteroids inhibit growth by stimulating production of somatomedin inhibitors. Characterization and improved assay of these factors may provide better insight into methods to circumvent their action.

Because the impairment in linear growth is directly dose related, it is important to use the lowest dose that will achieve the desired immunosuppressive effect. It has been established that less frequent administration, including alternate-day regimens, may mitigate or prevent deleterious effect on growth. Unterman and Phillips have demonstrated normal levels of somatomedin biologic activity in patients on the day off steroids when they are receiving alternate-day corticosteroid therapy.[4] Different corticosteroids (Table 1) have different relative potencies and, hence, also have varying effects on growth. The normal endogenous production of cortisol has been estimated to be 12–13 $mg/m^2/day$; by referring to Table 1, the "physiologic" equivalent of prednisone (4 $mg/m^2/day$) or other corticosteroids can be estimated. Such generalizations do not take into account the different half-life in plasma of the pharmaceutical derivatives when compared to cortisol, the physiologic corticosteroid secreted by the human adrenal gland.

In addition to suppression of growth, corticosteroid excess results in excessive weight gain and loss of muscle strength. They may induce impaired glucose tolerance or overt diabetes, probably by interfering with the action of insulin. Occasionally, emotional disturbances and even psychotic reactions may occur. Professionals who are managing children who have had cardiac transplantation should be alert to these side effects of corticosteroid excess and to utilize these agents judiciously. Eventually, pharmaceuticals having more specific effects on the immune response will replace corticosteroids with their myriad of undesirable effects.

Table 1. Relative Potencies of Steroids

	Glucocorticoid Activity	Mineralocorticoid Activity
Hydrocortisone	1	1
Cortisone	0.7	0.7
Prednisone	4	0.7
Prednisolone	4	0.7
Dexamethasone	30	2
Aldosterone	0.1	400
Fludrocortisone	10	400

References

1. Hyams JS, Carey DE: Corticosteroids and growth. J Pediatr 1988, 113: 249.
2. Strickland AL, Underwood LE, Voina SJ, et al: Growth retardation in Cushing's syndrome. Am J Dis Child 1972, 123:207.
3. Gourmelen M, Girard F, Binoux M: Serum somatomedin/insulin-like growth factor (IGF) and IGF carrier levels in patients with Cushing's syndrome or receiving glucocorticoid therapy. J Clin Endocrinol Metab 1982, 54:885.
4. Unterman TG, Phillips LS: Glucocorticoid effects of somatomedins and somatomedin inhibitors. J Clin Endocrinol Metab 1985, 61:518.

Chapter 11

Monitoring and Treatment of Rejection

Richard M. Donner and Bruce I. Goldman

The recognition and management of graft rejection remains a fundamental problem in the care of all cardiac allograft recipients. Following the introduction of cyclosporine A, clinical and pathologic findings suggested that it was useful to consider two forms of rejection, acute and chronic. This approach is based on well-recognized differences in timing, histology, and clinical manifestations between the two forms. Although we distinguish the two forms when establishing protocols and principles of treatment, further investigation into the cellular mechanisms of rejection and immunosuppression may demonstrate a close relationship between the two. It is possible, therefore, that our approach to the management of rejection will be altered significantly in the near future.

It is not prudent to assume that principles governing graft rejection in the adult are immediately applicable to the pediatric patient. Issues of recipient size, immunologic status, immunosuppressive effect, linear growth, and psychologic and social adjustment might influence the theoretical and practical strategies developed for adults. In recent years, a number of studies in comparatively small pediatric populations have drawn some parallels to the adult experience, but have also identified a number of differences, particularly in the new-

From *Heart Transplantation in Children,* edited by Jeffrey M. Dunn, M.D. and Richard M. Donner, M.D.

born. The data currently available are small but offer a foundation on which to construct a program for managing rejection.

Acute Rejection

The occurrence of at least one episode of acute rejection requiring treatment is a nearly universal finding in children following transplantation. In the presence of cyclosporine A with prednisone and/or azathioprine therapy, the number of rejections per patient averages 1.5 to 2.5 with a range of 0 to 5.[1–4] The great majority of these occur within the first 3 months after transplant. These data are obviously influenced by short-term follow-up in some patients and limited experience with pediatric heart transplantation in general. In terms of events per 100 patient-days, however, the results are similar, showing a steady decrease in the rate during the first 6 months postoperatively and only an occasional episode after 1 year.[1] Although patient numbers are fewer, it appears that newborn infants transplanted within the 1st month display the same phenomenon.[5] In children of any age, death from rejection does not seem to correlate with the number of early episodes or the time to first occurrence, but rather, from the severity of any one episode, the timing of therapy and response to treatment. The number, severity, and timing of rejection episodes in children do not differ significantly from findings in adult transplant recipients.[1,6]

It is generally agreed that any single method or combination of methods used to diagnose acute rejection must provide nearly 100% sensitivity and extremely high specificity. Of the two, sensitivity is more important because failure to diagnose acute rejection invariably leads to organ death. A fundamental axiom remains, "when in doubt, treat for rejection." The problem of specificity is more critical in the infant and young child in whom clinical signs of infection may be confused with those of rejection. Inappropriately augmented immunosuppression in the presence of some infectious processes is also life-threatening.

Endomyocardial Biopsy

Given the above considerations, there is little question that endomyocardial biopsy (EMB) is the diagnostic method of choice and also the standard by which other modalities (see below) are evaluated. In the older infant, young child, teenager, and adult, significant biopsy-proven rejection almost always precedes the clinical symptoms of fever, lethargy, palpitations, and signs of heart failure, such as tachycardia, tachypnea, gallop, venous distention, peripheral edema, and hepatomegaly.[2,3,7] In our own early series of 7 patients and 71 biopsies,[4] we observed 9 episodes of acute rejection unaccompanied by symptoms or abnormal physical examination and noninvasive testing. Only 2 of 13 biopsies performed for the presence of symptoms showed acute rejection. It is of great interest, however, that at least two centers performing neonatal transplants have successfully managed a number of infants without EMB. Very close clinical surveillance for fever, irritability, change in feeding habits, and signs of heart failure, along with laboratory and noninvasive testing, was responsible for the successful identification and treatment of acute rejection with no late deaths in either series.[5,8]

Biopsy Protocol

Routine EMB is scheduled frequently during the early postoperative months when the incidence of rejection is expected to be highest. Practical circumstances and rejection episodes may modify the schedule somewhat, but we try to adhere to the following: weekly for the first month, biweekly for the next 2 months, and monthly for the following 6 months. If acute rejection is no longer encountered, the frequency is gradually reduced to every 6 months. Each episode of rejection is followed by EMB approximately 10 days after initiating treatment to insure an adequate response. In nearly all cases, EMB is also performed if clinical manifestations of acute rejection, mentioned previously, are present. We prefer to use clinical judgment and have not developed a formal clinical scoring system. However, a new finding of palpitations or documented dysrhythmia is a very strong indication for EMB.

EMB is scheduled as an outpatient procedure, generally beginning very early in the morning to permit discharge in the early afternoon and the complete processing and interpretation of the specimen. Sedation is rarely used in children over 4 years of age. When required in younger children and infants, we have used a mixture of meperidine, promethazine, and chlorpromazine (2:1:1), administered intramuscularly.

Biopsy Procedure

Although transvenous EMB was first described in 1962,[9] the percutaneous approach and application to the diagnosis of acute rejection was made popular in 1973 by Caves et al.[10] The original technique was described in adults and utilized a rather inflexible bioptome passed through the internal jugular vein and into the right ventricle via the tricuspid valve. This technique remains applicable to nearly all adults, teenagers, and older children. The need for repetitive biopsy, the smaller vessel size, and psychological factors in newborns, infants, and younger children make this single approach difficult and impractical. To minimize complications and preserve vessel access, we and others utilize the femoral approach and a more flexible instrument.[11–13] When possible, the right and left femoral veins are used alternately. Careful attention to technique and a gentle approach are important to minimize scar tissue at the site, prevent thrombosis of the vessel, and insure easy, repeated access. At present, we select one of two biopsy forceps (Cordis Corp., Miami, FL, USA), a 5F, 75-cm instrument for infants and children under 4 years and a 5.4F, 104-cm instrument for older children. Both have a 2-mm specimen cup that usually yields adequate samples. The longer forceps has a central spring that insures closure of the cup if pressure on the handle is accidentally released. This feature also permits a gentle curve to be placed in the tip just adjacent to the hinge point of the specimen cup. However, it imparts a stiffness to the forceps that is not desirable in infants. The shorter forceps can be manufactured without this spring. Although no curve can be placed at the tip, its flexibility and ability to transmit the sensation of contact compare favorably to standard catheters when manipulated through a 6F sheath. The procedure itself begins by placing a 6F, 44-cm or 59-cm sheath with a 180° precurved tip (USCI, Billerica, MA, USA) in the inferior vena cava. The sheath should be matched (and occasionally trimmed) to the forceps to permit several centimeters of forceps to extend beyond the tip. A wedge pressure catheter is inserted through the sheath and positioned in the apex of the right ventricle. After obtaining hemodynamic data and appropriate laboratory blood samples, the sheath is advanced over the catheter into the midportion of the ventricle, and the catheter is removed. The biopsy forceps is then inserted until light contact is made and the specimen cup is closed (Fig. 1). An attempt is made to obtain three samples from different locations in children over 1 year and two sam-

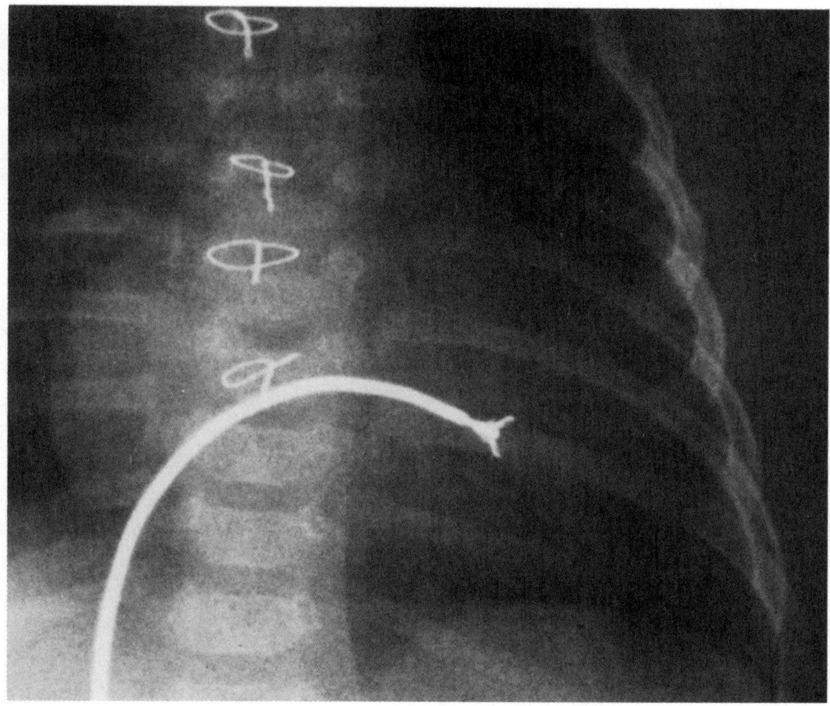

Figure 1: *Placement of a biopsy forceps in the right ventricle of a 5-month-old infant. The specimen cup is open. The forceps is positioned through a long sheath previously guided into the ventricle over a Swan-Ganz catheter.*

ples from infants. Care must be taken to eliminate all air from the sheath when removing and reinserting the forceps.

In our initial 71 biopsies (245 specimens), the procedure averaged 32 ± 15 minutes in length. We did not experience any clinical evidence of perforation, although three specimens contained small amounts of epicardial fat. One biopsy yielded insufficient tissue and was repeated on the afternoon of admission. In one autopsy specimen, the site of EMB performed 24 hours earlier was not apparent. Although neither we nor others have had experience with repeated EMB in newborn infants, the procedure seems to be feasible and safe in both infants and children.

Biopsy Interpretation

A discussion of the interpretation of endomyocardial biopsies in a symposium on pediatric cardiac transplantation is certainly appropriate, as EMB is recognized as an indispensable tool in the management of transplant recipients and the "gold standard" in the diagnosis of rejection.[10,14–17] Several excellent papers have already described the histopathology of EMB from the cardiac transplant recipient,[10,14–19] and the reader is referred to these for examples of typical histopathology and more thorough coverage of this topic. The purpose of this brief discussion is to summarize our current understanding of the clinical importance of certain patterns of biopsy histopathology in cardiac transplant recipients and to mention some problems peculiar to the interpretation of pediatric biopsies. In its course, this review will touch on some recent developments that have important implications concerning both the use of the EMB in diagnosis and management and our understanding of the pathobiology of the transplanted heart.

The primary use of EMB in the management of cardiac transplant recipients is in the diagnosis, grading, and post-treatment monitoring of acute cardiac rejection. Although different transplant centers may employ slightly different grading classification systems,[14–19] most acknowledge their basis in the work of Billingham, who first established a reproducible grading system with clear clinical applicability.[14,20] Simply stated, the Billingham system classifies acute rejection into mild, moderate, severe, and resolving grades based on the presence of subendocardial or perivascular lymphoid infiltrates (mild), infiltrates plus myocyte damage or necrosis (moderate), widespread necrosis with an infiltrate that also includes polymorphonuclears and hemorrhage (severe), and infiltrates composed primarily of macrophages and fibroblasts (resolving). These are illustrated in Figure 2. Application of this grading system is believed to be, in part, responsible for currently observed high post-transplant survival rates.[21]

One area of recent controversy, however, concerns the significance of subendocardial and perivascular lymphoid infiltrates in cyclosporine-treated recipients. In patients immunosuppressed without cyclosporine A, any such lymphoid infiltrate is taken as evidence of acute rejection requiring treatment; such infiltrates diminish with increased immunosuppression and progress in its absence.[7] Only a fraction of cyclosporine-treated patients with lymphoid infiltrates in their biopsies, however, will experience worsening rejection if left

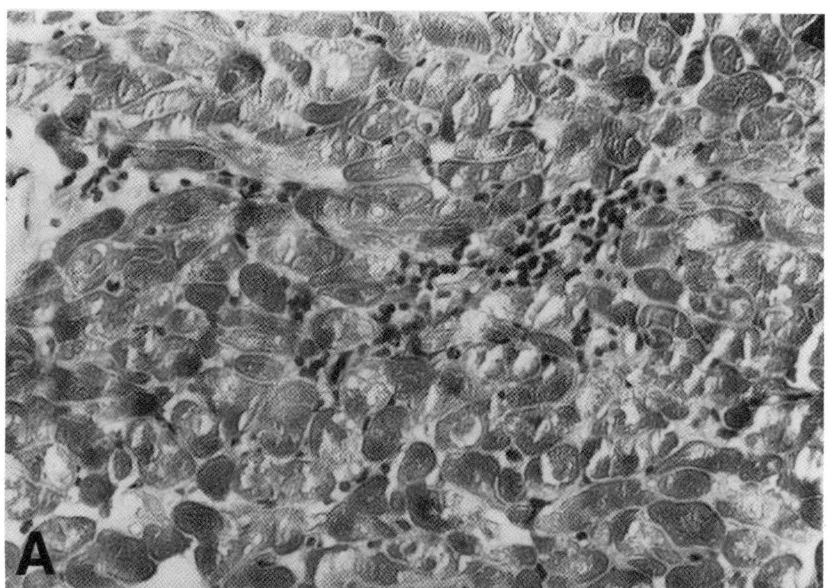

Figures 2A, B, C: *Photomicrographs showing typical histopathological appearance of mild (A, above), moderate (B), and severe (C) acute cardiac transplant rejection (hematoxylin and eosin stain, original magnification 75×.)*

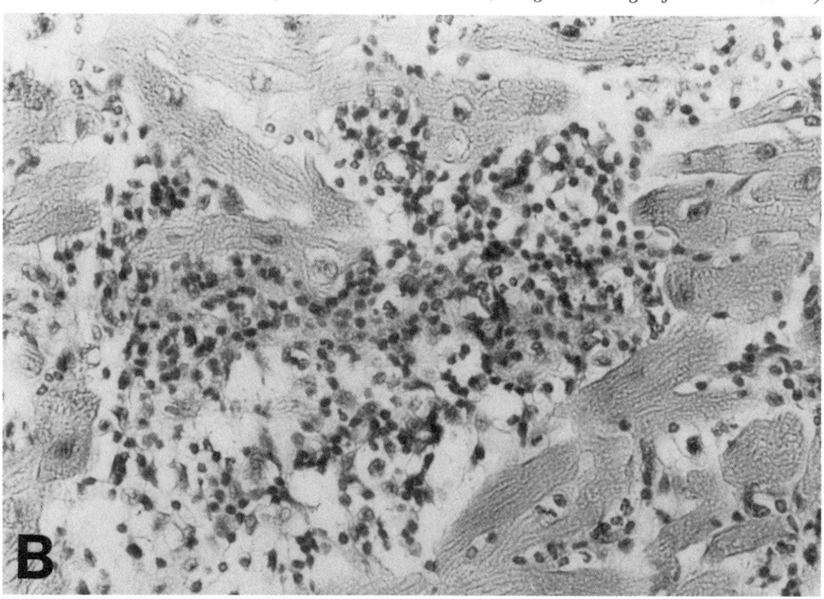

Figure 2B.

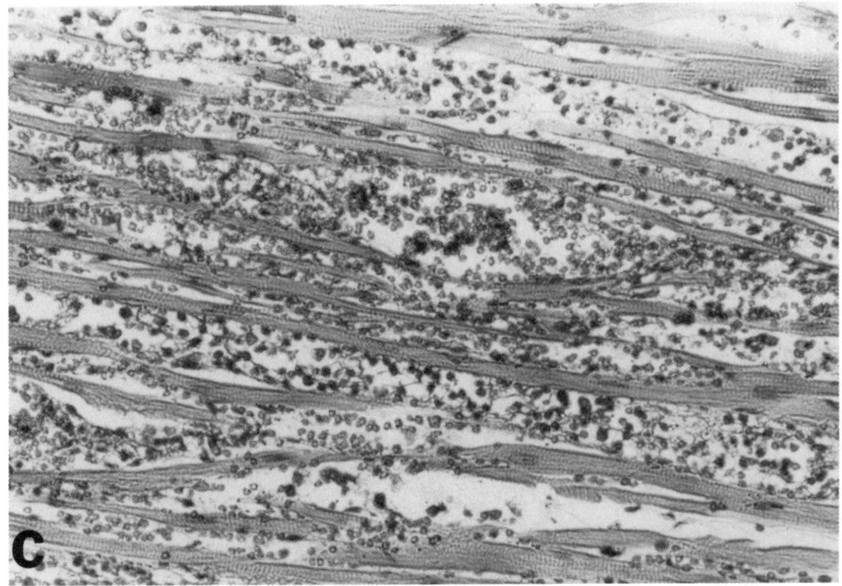

Figure 2C.

untreated.[22] It is not clear if this represents "arrested" rejection or a side effect of cyclosporine use, which is associated with the development of subendocardial and interstitial infiltrates.[14,15] Whatever the reason for this phenomenon, increased immunosuppression is generally not recommended for histologically mild acute rejection in patients receiving cyclosporine.[23] In the experience of Sibley et al.,[17] however, myocyte necrosis in EMB is a relatively rare finding, and even in cyclosporine-treated patients, infiltrates in the absence of necrosis may be accompanied by signs and symptoms of acute rejection. These authors employ a grading system based on this observation and recommend treatment for patients with "diffuse, intense" mononuclear infiltration, whether or not necrosis is present. Although their histologic criteria are somewhat subjective and thus may be difficult for others to apply, other studies have identified histologic features of lymphoid infiltration that appear to be predictive of progressing rejection in a significant proportion of patients and thus may be used as criteria for rebiopsy or treatment when infiltrates are not accompanied by myocyte necrosis or damage.[19,22] The predictive features identified in these studies are somewhat similar and include significant interstitial edema, extension of lymphoid infiltrate into the interstitial space between individual myocytes, and multifocal perivascular leukocytoclasis.[19,22] Some of these predictive features have been incorporated into a new classification system for EMB interpretation.[19]

Of course, the goal of all these various systems of interpretation is to most reliably minimize the occurrence of rejection episodes that damage the heart, while simultaneously minimizing the degree of required immunosuppression. The sensitivity and specificity of diagnostic tests are usually inversely related; however, any system that broadens the criteria for diagnosis of acute rejection requiring treatment will likely increase both the number of acute rejection episodes interrupted, as well as the number of patients treated unnecessarily. The increase in the former would likely be seen as a decrease in the frequency of significant rejection episodes per patient and may or may not have an impact on overall survival; increases in the latter might be seen as increased rates of infection, but might only be manifest as a decrease in quality of life for the patients, an effect difficult to identify or quantify. Ethics aside, it would seem that even a randomized trial comparing different classification systems might not really provide any definitive evidence as to which classification system is truly "the best." Thus, despite the effectiveness of EMB in the diagnosis and management of acute rejection, it is clear that an improved means of identifying acute rejection is still needed. The foregoing discussion is predicated, in part, on the assumption that moderate and severe rejection are particularly deleterious because, by definition, they result in irreversibly damaged myocytes. This assumption, which is based on light microscopic observations, has been challenged by Myles et al.[16] In an ultrastructural study of EMB from 45 patients, they found *no* ultrastructural evidence of irreversible damage, regardless of whether or not apparent necrosis was seen on light microscopy. Furthermore, the observed changes of myocyte damage also apparently reversed themselves with treatment. These authors argue that myocyte damage, and not necrosis per se, is the proper criterion for rejection that requires treatment and that treatment may frequently produce reversal of damage, with no permanent sequelae. Although the results of this study could reflect sampling error and do not provide an ultrastructural correlate of resolving rejection seen on light microscopy, theirs is still a finding worthy of further study, if only from the point of view of rejection pathobiology. As an extra benefit, their results also serve to remind us of the gulf that may exist between histopathology and biologic reality. Although Billingham's original grading system for acute rejection did not incorporate "vascular rejection" as an independent diagnostic criterion, some studies suggest that it may be informative to do so. Hershkowitz et al.[24] have identified acute arteriolitis as a histologic finding that may be difficult to distinguish from mild or moderate rejection, but one that is associated with early graft failure or dysfunction. Kemnitz et al.,[19] in their modification of the Billingham system, also include a category of "vasculopathy." Although their study does not specifically address the prognostic or therapeutic importance of acute arteriolitis, they do associate vasculopathy seen on biopsy with the presence of chronic rejection or "aggressive fibrosis."[19] Chronic rejection primarily affects the coronary arteries, producing intimal fibroproliferative lesions that may result in cardiac ischemia or infarction.[15] Such coronary artery disease constitutes a significant source of late morbidity and mortality in cardiac transplant recipients.[25] Identification of 13 intimal proliferative lesions in the small vessels seen on EMB thus probably represents a poor prognostic sign. In the author's experience, however, its absence may not be meaningful; in the autopsied heart of a patient who survived 5 years after transplantation, severe three-vessel coronary artery disease was present without concomitant disease of the intramural vessels. This tendency for chronic rejection to affect the epicardial coronary arteries preferentially has been noted by others.[15]

In addition to the histopathology changes associated with rejection, other histopathologic patterns often seen on EMB include those attributed to ischemia, previous biopsy, infection, cyclosporine use (alluded to earlier), and more rarely, malignancy. The histologic characteristics of these lesions have been well described by Pomerance et al.[15] In general, the presence of any of them does not usually pose serious diagnostic problems, although it is wise for the reviewing pathologist to have a reasonably high index of suspicion for them. Still, nonrejection pathology may be relatively more important in pediatric EMB because those processes that tend to be located subendocardially (e.g., cyclosporine-associated infiltrates and previous biopsy effect) will be disproportionally represented in the small, more superficial biopsies obtained from pediatric patients and thus may be more likely to mask the changes of acute rejection. Additionally, previous biopsy sites are more prone to repeated sampling in smaller hearts and thus would be expected to be seen more frequently on EMB. These factors may decrease the sensitivity of EMB in the diagnosis of rejection in pediatric patients. Related to this issue is the question of biopsy sample size as a determinant of diagnostic sensitivity. Studies in adults have shown that three or four pieces obtained with a 9F bioptome provide adequate tissue for reasonable (95%–98%) sensitivity in the diagnosis of acute rejection.[26] Although we generally assume that the same rule applies proportionally to smaller biopsies obtained from smaller hearts, this assumption has not been tested. Criteria for determining adequacy of sample size in pediatric patients thus remain unestablished. The already mentioned tendency for previous biopsy sites and cyclosporine-associated infiltrates to be disproportionally represented in small biopsies only serves to complicate this question.

This brief review has attempted to summarize what we know (and do not know) concerning the clinical implications of certain histopathologic changes found in EMB from cardiac transplant recipients and to discuss some problems peculiar to pediatric biopsies. As has been mentioned earlier, however, our interpretation of biopsies from pediatric patients largely assumes that the histopathology (and by inference the biologic behavior) of pediatric transplants is essentially identical to that of adult allografts. There is no intrinsic reason why this should necessarily be true; in fact, there are numerous examples in other contexts where it clearly is not. With the increasing success of cardiac transplantation as a viable mode of therapy for pediatric patients with end-stage heart disease, it should be possible—and indeed is necessary—to evaluate the use and interpretation of EMB specifically in the pediatric transplant population.

Noninvasive Methods

The current rationale for developing noninvasive methods to detect acute allograft rejection in pediatric transplant recipients is twofold: (1) to eliminate or reduce the number of biopsy procedures, especially in newborns and infants; and (2) to establish the need for EMB as a nonscheduled procedure between routinely scheduled biopsies. The extent to which either or both of these rationales are observed depends upon the experience and philosophy of the transplant team. In most centers, a comfortable compromise will be made using age and ease of venous access as criteria; it is more likely that acute rejection will be treated on the basis of noninvasive evaluation in an infant than in an older child. Because exhaustive studies of individual noninvasive methods have not been performed in the pediatric population, much over-diagnosis and treatment will and should occur to avoid graft loss.

The principle noninvasive modalities are surface electrocardiography, intramyocardial electrograms, echocardiography, nuclear magnetic resonance, and radioimmunodetection.

Surface Electrocardiography

In the absence of acute rejection, the surface electrocardiogram in the cardiac allograft recipient differs from a normal tracing. Recipient and donor P waves are identified in many. The resting heart rate in adults is increased to between 95 and 115 beats/min in the absence of vagal innervation and nonspecific T wave changes are common.[27] In the presence of EMB proven rejection (myocyte necrosis), the sum of scalar voltages in leads I, II, and III, plus those of selected precordial leads (usually V_1 and V_6), decreases in comparison with a "baseline" reference determined in the absence of rejection.[27,28] A reduction of voltage by 20% over a 24-hour period is typical of criteria suggested for the diagnosis of moderate rejection.[27] Problems with this method include poor sensitivity and specificity, progressive reduction of the "baseline" summed voltage due to repeated rejection, and the appearance of voltage reduction several days after the onset of cell destruction.[7,27–29] It has been suggested that signal averaging may improve the sensitivity and specificity of ECG monitoring in adults.[28] Although dysrhythmias were not a major feature of rejection in most adult series, we have noticed an increased frequency of atrial and ventricular extrasystoles in some patients, whereas others never exhibit this phenomenon during rejection. However, an increase in resting heart rate is observed in the majority of our patients. Most ECG manifestations of rejection disappear with successful treatment.

Intramyocardial Electrogram

With pacemaker technology that offers waveform telemetry, it is now possible to examine isolated and summed intramyocardial electrograms. The right ventricular electrogram was examined in adults by Warnecke et al.[30] Changes in voltage reflected the presence of moderate rejection with 88% sensitivity and 96% specificity. No similar studies have been performed in children, however, and caution has been suggested regarding diurnal variation of voltage.[31] The necessity of implanting a pacemaker also has disadvantages for the pediatric population.

Echocardiography

In both adults and children, simple assessment of left ventricular ejection and pump function (ejection fraction, shortening fraction, ejection time) does not distinguish the presence of mild or moderate acute rejection in cyclosporine-treated patients.[29,32,33] Severe rejection is often accompanied by physical signs of heart failure and depression of pump function as assessed by any method. The mechanics of diastolic filling are affected by acute rejection (EMB) in children and adults as evidenced by the shortening of isovolumic contraction time determined by ECG and M-mode echocardiography and by reduction of pressure half-time determined by Doppler echocardiography.[1,29,32,33] Like summated ECG voltage, these usually return to baseline values with successful treatment. Sensitivity, specificity and predictive values vary among the published studies, but are usually between 60% and 90%, significantly higher than for surface ECG monitoring. Baseline differences between transplanted and native hearts, the frequent occurrence of recipient–donor size mismatch, variations of ischemic time and donor heart viability, and progressive, nonuniform wall hypertrophy of the donor heart make absolute criteria for these indices more difficult to establish than is possible with some structural and functional heart disease. Therefore, nonrejection profiles in each recipient should be established for each index of diastolic performance.

The association of acute rejection in cyclosporine-treated patients and the presence of myocardial edema suggests that ultrasound image analysis may be used to detect rejection. Analysis of pixel brightness in static[34] and dynamic[35] images has been performed in animal models not treated with cyclosporine, but has not been applied to a pediatric population.

Nuclear Magnetic Resonance

Magnetic resonance imaging and spectroscopy have been examined as a tool for predicting acute rejection. NMR phosphorus spectroscopy in untreated animals has shown a decrease in phosphocreatine with mild and moderate rejection.[36] T2 relaxation time in treated, nonrejecting animals[37] and a small group of adults and children[38] does not differ from native hearts, but is elevated in the presence of acute rejection and correlates with the severity. Like analysis of ultrasound backscatter, this phenomenon is related to the presence of myocardial edema.

Radioimmunodetection

In a group of 17 adults and 1 child, indium-labeled antimyosin (Fab) antibody uptake yielded an 80% sensitivity, specificity, and predictive value for identifying the presence of moderate or severe rejection.[39] Further studies in children are needed to confirm its usefulness, but its application may be limited by the total amount of radiation delivered over a relatively short period of time.

Monoclonal antibodies to T lymphocytes (OKT series, Ortho Diagnostic Systems, Raritan, N.J., U.S.A.) may be used to detect populations of lymphocytes related to cell damage. A number of studies have investigated these populations, especially the T helper to T suppressor cytotoxic ratio (T4/T8). In a mixed group of adult and pediatric cardiac transplant recipients, the ratio rises just prior to the rejection process.[40] However, other factors such as infection may influence this. Further studies of this and other lymphocyte groups in pediatric patients are necessary.

Each of these noninvasive methods requires a minimum level of expertise and a specific familiarity with their applications to heart transplantation. At present, comparison of these methods with EMB yields sensitivities and specificities that vary widely among institutions. It is recommended that each institution establish specific familiarity with one or more methods and investigate the use of the individual patient as a control.

It must be remembered that each noninvasive method attempts to monitor a different component of the rejection process and may not reflect EMB findings in all circumstances. As immunosuppression and treatment of rejection evolve, one or more of these methods may replace EMB as the "gold standard."

Treatment of Acute Rejection

The appearance of symptoms in most disease states usually implies inadequate drug therapy. Unlike most conventional diseases, however, the appearance of moderate acute rejection does not necessarily mean that chronic immunosuppression is inadequate. Although the relation between acute and chronic rejection is not fully understood, episodes of moderate rejection are usually treated as separate entities, not requiring a change in chronic immunosuppression unless laboratory assay reveals inadequate blood concentrations. It is generally agreed that the most important indication for treatment of rejection is the presence or suspicion of moderate or severe acute rejection. Mild rejection, as defined above, is generally not treated because it usually does not progress to acute cell necrosis. A diagnosis of moderate or severe rejection is legitimately made by clinical grounds alone (in the case of neonates and young infants), by clinical suspicion supported by noninvasive testing and/or EMB, or by routinely scheduled EMB. A second indication for treatment is the presence of progressive, mild acute rejection present on EMB. A third indication is an inadequate response to previous treatment as determined by EMB (preferably) or by clinical or noninvasive means.

Treatment of moderate acute rejection implies the administration of one or more immunosuppressive agents in addition to the ongoing chronic immunosuppressive regimen.[1–3,5,6] Although protocols vary among institutions, pulsed steroids are usually the first drug of choice. Intravenous methylprednisolone, 10–20 mg/kg given over 1 to 3 hours on each of 3 days is a common choice. This intravenous regimen is utilized before discharge and sometimes extended for several weeks or months. We prefer to administer methylprednisolone up to 3 months posttransplant and have had little trouble arranging intravenous home administration. After this period, treatment consists of 1 mg/kg of oral prednisone for 3 to 5 days, followed by slow tapering to zero. If prednisone is part of chronic immunosuppression, this pulse is added to it and is tapered to the chronic dose over 1 to 2 weeks. Although a second course of intravenous steroids is often given if the biopsy-proven response is inadequate, some centers prefer to use 3 to 5 days of antithymocyte globulin (ATG), alone or with continuation of the steroids. OKT3, originally formulated as a diagnostic tool, can be used as a therapeutic agent and has been substituted for ATG, especially when the latter is in short supply. Severe rejection is usually treated with an initial course of methylprednisolone and ATG (10 mg/kg/day I.V. over 4 to 6 hours) for 3 to 5 days. Afterload reduction, diuretics, and inotropic agents may be necessary if heart failure is present. Often, prednisone will be added to the chronic immunosuppression if not already present, especially if pump function is impaired. Follow-up EMB may be scheduled a few days after starting treatment. We prefer to wait 7 to 10 days, however, in order to differentiate ongoing moderate rejection from resolving rejection. In young infants in whom EMB cannot be performed, resolution of the clinical symptoms (e.g., fussiness, poor feeding, fever, etc.) and/or return of noninvasive indices to normal constitutes proof of successful treatment.

Chronic Rejection

The major manifestation of chronic allograft rejection is severe coronary artery disease. This is accompanied by sequelae normally associated with this phenomenon: ischemia, loss of myocardium, and impaired cardiac performance. Typical anginal pain is not usually present in the denervated heart. Although chronic rejection is a significant source of morbidity and mortality in adults,[41] it is less known in children. Fricker et al.[3] discussed three children, ages 6, 8, and 13, with severe coronary disease 8 months after transplantation. One child died with chronic rejection, another with acute and chronic rejection, and the third required retransplantation for chronic rejection; death followed the development of rapid chronic rejection in the second organ. We have not experienced chronic rejection of this severity, especially so early in the clinical course. A recent preliminary review of serial coronary angiograms in seven of our patients demonstrated noticeable small vessel narrowing in only one patient 4 ½ years after transplant. It is likely that additional reports will follow in the near future. Whether this phenomenon will be a major source of morbidity and mortality in children, as it is in adults, remains unclear.

The preoperative evaluation of the potential recipient should reflect concern for the process of accelerated coronary artery disease. Because adults transplanted for severe coronary disease show a higher incidence of chronic rejection,[27] it is wise to obtain total plasma cholesterol, HDL cholesterol fraction, and triglycerides as part of pretransplant laboratory screening. Because chronic heart failure and a debilitated general state may affect these results, a prior lipid determination (if available) and family history of coronary artery disease are valuable.

The diagnosis of chronic rejection following transplant is based upon a continued suspicion, because symptoms may be few and sudden death may occur. The presence of intimal coronary fibrosis in routine EMB specimens should, of course, be noted and followed. Because this may not reflect the presence of large vessel disease, it is our practice to perform coronary angiography at least once each year (at the time of routinely scheduled EMB). In most children, vessels may be injected selectively, allowing a detailed comparison with previous angiograms. Lipid profiles are performed twice a year. Stress testing and stress thallium studies may also prove to identify the onset of significant coronary artery involvement.

Prophylactic treatment of chronic rejection has not been studied in detail. We review the importance of diet with each recipient family and make practical suggestions in accord with published recommendations.[42] We have not needed to supplement diet with a bile acid sequestrant (cholestyramine), but this remains a viable option, if required. An HMG-CoA reductase inhibitor (Lovastatin) has been used in a child who underwent combined heart and hepatic receptor site transplantation.[43] The prophylactic use of salicylates and omega-3 fatty acids in children needs to be addressed but may be considered in the presence of documented coronary artery involvement.

References

1. Starnes VA, Stinson EB, Oyer PE, et al: Cardiac transplantation in children and adolescents. Circulation 1987, 76(Suppl V):43.
2. Addonizio LJ, Rose EA: Cardiac transplantation in children and adolescents. J Pediatr 1987, 111:1034.
3. Fricker FJ, Griffith BP, Hardesty RL, et al: Experience with heart transplantation in children. Pediatrics 1987, 79:138.
4. Bhargava H, Donner RM, Sanchez G, et al: Endomyocardial biopsy after heart transplantation in children. J Heart Transplant 1987, 6:298.
5. Mavroudis C, Harrison H, Klein JB, et al: Infant orthotopic cardiac transplantation. J Thorac Cardiovasc Surg 1988, 96:912.
6. Dunn JM, Cavarocchi NS, Balsara RK: Pediatric heart transplantation at St. Christopher's Hospital for Children. J Heart Transplant 1987, 6:334.

7. Caves PK, Stinson EB, Billingham ME, et al: Serial transvenous biopsy of the transplanted human heart. Improved management of acute rejection episodes. Lancet 1974, i:821.
8. Bailey LL, Assaad AN, Trim RF, et al: Orthotopic transplantation during infancy as therapy for incurable congenital heart disease. Ann Surg 1988, 208:279.
9. Sakakibara S, Konno S: Endomyocardial biopsy. Jpn Heart J 1962, 3:537.
10. Caves PK, Stinson EB, Billingham M, et al: Percutaneous transvenous endomyocardial biopsy in human heart recipients. Experience with a new technique. Ann Thorac Surg 1973, 4:325.
11. Lurie PR, Fujita M, Neustein HB: Transvascular endomyocardial biopsy in infants and small children. Am J Cardiol 1978, 42:453.
12. Anderson JL, Marshall HW, Allison SB: The femoral venous approach to endomyocardial biopsy: Comparison with internal jugular and transarterial approaches. Am J Cardiol 1984, 53:833.
13. De Moor MMA, Human DG: Endomyocardial biopsy technique in infants and small children. S Afr Med J 1984, 69:439.
14. Billingham ME: Diagnosis of cardiac rejection by endomyocardial biopsy. Heart Transplant 1982, 1:25.
15. Pomerance A, Stovin PGI: Heart transplant pathology: The British experience. J Clin Pathol 1985, 38:146.
16. Myles JL, Ratliff NB, McMahon TJ, et al: Reversibility of myocyte injury in moderate and severe acute rejection in cyclosporine-treated cardiac transplant patients. Arch Pathol Lab Med 1987, 111:947.
17. Sibley RK, Olivari MT, Bolman RM, et al: Endomyocardial biopsy in the cardiac allograft recipient: A review of 570 biopsies. Ann Surg 1986, 203: 177.
18. McAllister H Jr, Schnee MJ, Radovancevic B, et al: A system for grading cardiac allograft rejection. Texas Heart Inst J 1986, 13:1.
19. Kemnitz J, Cohnert T, Schafers HJ, et al: A classification of cardiac allograft rejection: A modification of the classification by Billingham. Am J Surg Pathol 1987, 11:503.
20. Caves PK, Stinson EB, Billingham ME, et al: Diagnosis of human cardiac allograft rejection by serial cardiac biopsy. J Thorac Cardiovasc Surg 1973, 66:461.
21. Billingham ME: (letter) Ann Surg 1986, 204:725.
22. Hershkowitz A, Soule LM, Mellits ED, et al: Histologic predictors of acute cardiac rejection in human endomyocardial biopsies: A multivariate analysis. J Am Coll Cardiol 1987, 9:802.
23. Billingham ME: Endomyocardial detection of acute rejection in cardiac allograft recipients. Heart Vessels 1985, 1(Suppl I):86.
24. Hershkowitz A, Soule LM, Veda K, et al: Arteriolar vasculitis on endomyocardial biopsy: A histologic prediction of poor outcome in cyclosporine-treated heart transplant recipients. J Heart Transplant 1987, 6:127.
25. Kaye MP: The registry of the International Society for Heart Transplantation: Fourth official report. 1987. J Heart Transplant 1987, 6:63.

26. Spiegelhalter DJ, Stovin PGI: An analysis of repeated biopsies following cardiac transplantation. Stat Med 1983,2:33.
27. Hess ML, Hastillo A, Wolfgang TC, et al: The noninvasive diagnosis of acute and chronic cardiac allograft rejection. Heart Transplant 1981, 1: 31.
28. Keren A, Gillis AM, Freedman RA, et al: Heart transplant rejection monitored by signal-averaged electrocardiography in patients receiving cyclosporine. Circulation 1984, 70(Suppl I):124.
29. Dawkins K, Oldershaw PJ, Billingham M, et al: Changes in diastolic function as a noninvasive marker of cardiac allograft rejection. Heart Transplant 1984, 3:286.
30. Warnecke H, Schuler S, Goetze H-J, et al: Noninvasive monitoring of cardiac allograft rejection by intramyocardial electrogram recordings. Circulation 1986, 74(Suppl III):72.
31. Wahlers T, Haverich A, Schafers K, et al: Changes of the intramyocardial electrogram after orthotopic heart transplantation. J Heart Transplant 1986, 5:450.
32. Valantine HA, Fowler MB, Hunt SA, et al: Changes in Doppler echocardiographic indexes of left ventricular function as potential markers of acute cardiac rejection. Circulation 1987, 76(Suppl V):86.
33. Desruennes M, Corcos T, Cabrol A, et al: Doppler echocardiography for the diagnosis of acute cardiac allograft rejection. J Am Coll Cardiol 1988, 12:63.
34. Chandrasekaran K, Bansal RC, Greenleaf JF, et al: Early recognition of heart transplant rejection by backscatter analysis from serial 2D echos in a heterotopic transplant model. J Heart Transplant 1987, 6:1.
35. Wear KA, Schnittger I, Director BA, et al: Ultrasonic characterization of acute cardiac rejection from temporal evolution of echocardiograms. J Heart Transplant 1986, 5:425.
36. Hall TS, Baumgartner WA, Borkon AM, et al: Diagnosis of acute cardiac rejection with antimyosin monoclonal antibody, phosphorus nuclear magnetic resonance imaging, two-dimensional echocardiography, and endocardial biopsy. J Heart Transplant 1986, 5:419.
37. Aherne T, Tscholakoff D, Finkbeiner W, et al: Magnetic resonance imaging of cardiac transplants: The evaluation of rejection of cardiac allografts with and without immunosuppression. Circulation 1986, 74:145.
38. Lund G, Morin RL, Olivari MT, et al: Serial myocardial T2 relaxation time measurements in normal subjects and heart transplant recipients. J Heart Transplant 1988, 7:274.
39. Frist W, Yasuda T, Segall G, et al: Noninvasive detection of human cardiac transplant rejection with indium-111 antimyosin (Fab) imaging. Circulation 1987, 76(Suppl V):81.
40. Hoshinaga K, Mohanakumar T, Pascoe EA, et al: Expression of transferrin receptors on lymphocytes: Its correlation with T-helper/T-suppressor cytotoxic ratio and rejection in heart transplant recipients. J Heart Transplant 1988, 7:198.

41. Uretsky BF, Murali S, Reddy PS, et al: Development of coronary artery disease in cardiac transplant patients receiving immunosupressive therapy with cyclosporine and prednisone. Circulation 1987, 76:827.
42. Weidman W, Kwiterovitch P, Jesse MJ, et al: Diet in the healthy child: Report of the Task Force Committee of the Nutrition Committee and the Cardiovascular Disease in the Young Council of the American Heart Association. Circulation 1983, 67:1411A.
43. East C, Grundy SM, Bilheimer DW: Normal cholesterol levels with Lovastatin (Mevinolin) therapy in a child with homozygous familial hypercholesterolemia following liver transplantation. JAMA 1986, 256:2843.

Chapter 12

Management of the Transplant Patient at Home: Practical Issues

Carolyn Vieweg

Management of the pediatric heart transplant recipient after discharge must deal with many of the same problems common to all children with significant congenital heart disease. To many of these children and their families, alterations of lifestyle are nothing new and may be taken for granted. However, the uniqueness of the procedure, its special medical requirements, and the tremendous health benefits achieved require that certain protocols be established. We have found that the teaching of these protocols and their integration into the family environment require a large commitment of time from the medical team, a requirement that often cannot be met satisfactorily. It is our experience that a full-time transplant coordinator is necessary to ensure that the benefits of the transplant procedure are fully realized.

General Considerations

Communication among the child and family, the transplant team, and the child's pediatrician is of great importance, because no other aspect of care can be successful without this. Communication begins

From *Heart Transplantation in Children*, edited by Jeffrey M. Dunn, M.D. and Richard M. Donner, M.D. © 1990, Futura Publishing Company, Inc., Mount Kisco, NY.

prior to discharge, when the transplant coordinator is linked with the family as all begin to review the essential components of home care. The family is instructed that contact with the transplant team is performed through the transplant coordinator and that this person is available at all times to perform necessary functions (Table 1). The transplant coordinator usually initiates communication with the family within the first 24 hours after discharge to answer questions, as well as to evaluate the level of understanding and confidence with home care. The contact continues on a weekly basis or as required until an acceptable level of confidence and performance is achieved. During the first few months following transplant, a close bond is established with the transplant coordinator, who assumes many of the functions of the traditional doctor–patient relationship. We have found this to be of great benefit and have only experienced family disturbances when a new coordinator was introduced to the transplant team.

Although child and family education begins prior to discharge, there is a continuing need to reinforce and update materials and instructions. Extensive written information is distributed to the family regarding the medications, their side effects, and dosages. We require that two bottles of cyclosporine be available at all times and that, in the case of infants and young children, at least two family members have experience in its administration. Instructions are given regarding the procedures to follow if a dose of medication is accidentally omitted or delayed. Once daily medications (e.g., azathioprine) are given in the

Table 1. Functions of the Transplant Coordinator

Preoperative
Introduction to family
Attend conferences with family
Arrange for all required laboratory testing and record results
Maintain contact during waiting period
Postoperative
Predischarge teaching
Initiate phone contact during first week and maintain as necessary
Arrange elective or emergency admissions as required
Arrange outpatient clinical and laboratory evaluations
Obtain, record, and report inpatient and outpatient laboratory data to transplant team
Inform family of medication changes
Maintain contact with pediatrician and other medical consultants
Arrange for outside agency involvement, if necessary (with social service)

evening to permit dose changes to be communicated to the family during the day. A relationship is established with a pharmacy that is able to obtain and provide refills of all medications and appropriate syringes or droppers without delay. The family is encouraged to assume responsibility for reporting changes in health. We emphasize that the following require contact with the coordinator: fever or other signs of infection, pain, irritability, poor appetite, lethargy, weight loss, vomiting, palpitations. The family understands that the transplant team will make whatever recommendations are necessary and will try to avoid inpatient care whenever possible. During the initial months after discharge, all symptoms are usually reported to the coordinator, but contact of this kind almost always diminishes as the patient and family become more comfortable with transient symptoms of intercurrent illness. Although we adhere to protocol guidelines whenever possible, our instructions must conform to the unique needs and abilities of individual families.

The need for communication among the family, transplant coordinator, and all members of the transplant team is satisfied by a weekly transplant conference that is organized and run by the coordinator and attended by key representatives of medical and surgical personnel. The coordinator assembles, records, and reports the status of each patient, including recent laboratory values, such as hemoglobin concentration, white blood cell count, routine chemistries, cyclosporine level, and endomyocardial biopsy. Social and practical issues are also discussed. Recommendations are made by the team regarding medication changes, repetition of laboratory tests, and scheduling of routine endomyocardial biopsy. A discussion of all accepted and potential transplant candidates is also held and the status of each, as well as the progress of the pretransplant evaluation, is determined and recorded. The coordinator is then responsible for contacting appropriate families and making all necessary arrangements.

During the 6 to 12 months after transplant, virtually all of the child's medical care is assumed by the transplant team. This is reasonable, because day-to-day problems, such as intercurrent illnesses, assume greater significance and require familiarity and expertise to deal with them correctly and efficiently. Although the pediatrician or family physician will not play an active role at this time, it is vital that this individual be kept informed of the child's progress so there will be a willingness to assume much of the routine care at a later date. Some direct contact between the pediatrician and the transplant team should occur, but we have found that occasional phone calls (approximately once each month) and written summaries to the pediatrician from the transplant coordinator are greatly appreciated and are effective in establishing a system of routine child care for the future. These communications should contain not only a summary of recent events but also information regarding routine immunization, restrictions of activity (if any), problems of social adjustment, and precautions to be taken during the course of everyday activities. In some cases, the transplant coordinator becomes the most important resource for the pediatrician and maintains a major portion of the contact.

A variety of nursing and home care services may be employed to reduce the number of inpatient admissions and outpatient visits. Medications such as intravenous methylprednisolone may be administered in the home without difficulty and frequent laboratory blood samples, which must be obtained in the early morning, may be drawn locally and brought to the medical center without disturbing the school schedule. Community agencies, local governments, and nonprofit institutions may also be called upon to assist the patient's family with their financial burden. This is important, to assure that medication is not interrupted and that anxiety is reduced to a minimum. Other services frequently available are psychosocial counseling and transportation. Involvement of the social service worker is critical if all of these needs are to be filled in an efficient manner. This individual also maintains close contact with the family, when appropriate, and attends the weekly transplant conference regularly.

Special Considerations

Infection Precautions

During hospitalization, the child remains in a private room isolated from other children who may be carrying potentially threatening infections. At the time of discharge, however, integration into a normal environment begins and all isolation is removed. For example, the child may continue to share a room with a sibling. It is not practical to completely isolate the child from infectious disease within the family, but we encourage family members who have a potentially communicable respiratory illness to avoid direct contact with the child if possible. If this is not feasible, then strict handwashing by all and the wearing of a mask by the affected individual are recommended. Family members and friends from outside the household are asked not to visit if they are ill, and visitors to the home should be screened for infectious disease and communicable disease exposure. It is probably wise to maintain the home in a general state of cleanliness, but adjustments such as removing pets are unnecessary. To permit medical care to be as uncomplicated as possible during the first few weeks after discharge, it has been our custom to delay the return to school or day care setting for 1 month and to prohibit the child from exposure to large crowds. After this period, these activities and others that place the child in close contact with well individuals (such as sleeping overnight at a friend's home) are permitted and encouraged. If a large outbreak of a disease such as chicken pox, measles, or strep throat has developed in the school after the child's return, it is recommended that he stay home during this outbreak.

It has been our experience that transplant recipients do not develop respiratory illness more frequently than their normal peers. The majority of intercurrent respiratory tract disease is handled well and resolves within a few days. During the first few months following transplant, even mild respiratory illness will evoke some concern by the transplant team and often lead to a brief outpatient visit and laboratory studies. With the passage of time, however, such symptoms may go unreported or may not require medical attention if they are mild and self limited.

Return to School and Physical Activity

Aside from the 1-month period we impose to minimize early infectious complications, reentry into the school environment is a function of physical recovery from surgery. Participation in the physical education program is often delayed for 2 or 3 months to reduce the possibility of serious trauma to the chest and sternum. Despite differences in regulation of cardiac function, many of our older children and teenagers have demonstrated normal or superior athletic ability, and we encourage full participation in the physical education program and permit them to take part in strenuous, competitive interscholastic sports.

Three other factors may combine to complicate the reentry process. Although the child thinks of himself as physically and mentally normal, the significant school time missed because of the prior illness may result in placement one or more grades below former classmates. Alternatively, a great deal of remedial work may be necessary to maintain a position in the former grade level. A second problem we have encountered is the natural reluctance on the part of school staff to integrate the child into routine activities as quickly as possible. A third obstacle is the planned or unanticipated school time lost for outpatient visits, laboratory work, and endomyocardial biopsy. All of these problems need to be addressed by parents, administrators, and guidance personnel prior to the actual date of return. It has been our practice for the transplant coordinator to contact parents and school officials in order to raise these issues in a timely fashion, to offer a written summary of the child's prognosis and special needs, and to stress the importance of normalizing the child's school environment and experiences. On occasion, a visit to the school has been necessary to review the child's status with the nurse and/or principal. Relationships made with school officials at this time avoid problems if recommendations have to be altered at a later date.

Most children who have undergone heart transplant return to school in much better physical condition and their class participation and performance improve greatly. As pediatric transplantation becomes more common and information is routinely disseminated to educators, difficulties involving school reentry should become less frequent.

Travel

If the initial course has been smooth, short trips out of the immediate area are encouraged. Because acute rejection is a medical emergency, more distant traveling requires good planning and the establishment of reliable telephone communication. On one occasion, we coordinated a vacation trip with a transplant center close to the vacation site.

Emotional Status of the Child and Family

As the child begins his recovery from transplant surgery, a number of problems may arise. Prior to transplant, the gravely ill child may exhibit feelings of isolation and depression. Following transplant surgery, we have noted a state of euphoria and frequent mood swings in several children during the postoperative hospitalization, a finding exaggerated by the administration of steroids to treat acute rejection. A similar, but less marked euphoria may be observed in the parents as they witness a "miraculous" change in their child's state of health. This reaction to the new state of well-being seems to be self-limited in both child and parent as both return to a more normal lifestyle during the first few months after discharge. Wishing to maintain a favorable recovery, however, some parents will resist efforts to remove the protective care and close surveillance established in the postoperative period. The first overnight stay with a friend or trip to a crowded movie theater can be a traumatic experience for parents, but it is this form of independence and responsibility that must be encouraged by the transplant team and family members. It is important for all who care for the family and child to anticipate and recognize these patterns of behavior in order to counter them more effectively.

Chapter 13

Infections and Immunizations

Margaret C. Fisher

Infections remain a major cause of morbidity and mortality in recipients of organ transplants.[1–4] The type of infection depends on the environment and the host. The major host factor is the extent of immunosuppression.[5–8]

Children with congenital or acquired heart disease are often at increased risk for infection even before transplantation. Furthermore, many do not receive the usual childhood immunizations. This chapter reviews immunization and infection of the heart transplant recipient; it is divided into pretransplantation, peritransplantation, and posttransplantation periods.

Pretransplantation

Children with heart failure are predisposed to infection for a variety of reasons. Pulmonary edema interferes with normal lung defenses. The enlarged heart causes atelectasis of segments of lung by compression of the bronchi.[9] Malnutrition occurs in some children with chronic heart failure; one consequence of malnutrition is immunosuppression.[10,11] Children with end-stage heart disease are frequently hospitalized and receive multiple courses of antibiotics. Severe illness alone alters normal flora. Studies of patients hospitalized in intensive care units show that normal oropharyngeal flora is re-

From *Heart Transplantation in Children,* edited by Jeffrey M. Dunn, M.D. and Richard M. Donner, M.D. © 1990, Futura Publishing Company, Inc., Mount Kisco, NY.

placed by enteric gram-negative bacilli.[12] Antibiotic therapy further alters flora and selects for colonization by resistant organisms. Invasive procedures, indwelling catheters, and mechanical ventilation increase the risk of nosocomial infections.[13]

Infections during the pretransplantation period are both community and hospital acquired. Little can be done to prevent many community-acquired illnesses. Immunization plays a major role in prevention of several serious infections. Many children with chronic disease do not receive the recommended immunizations because the parents or primary physician feel that the child is "too sick" to be vaccinated.[14] This attitude must be changed.[15] The opportunity to fully immunize a child is prior to transplantation. The usual vaccines, oral polio vaccine (OPV), diphtheria-tetanus-pertussis (DPT), measles-mumps-rubella (MMR), and *Haemophilus influenzae* type B (HIB), should be given (Table 1). If immunizations have been delayed, the schedule shown in Table 2 should be started. If the patient has an immunologic deficiency (e.g., DiGeorge syndrome) or is receiving immunosuppressive therapy, routine immunizations are not given.[16] Live vaccines (OPV and MMR) should be avoided if transplantation is anticipated in the near future. If transplantation can be safely delayed, then immunization should be completed prior to the procedure.

In addition to these routine immunizations, immunization against influenza, pneumococci, and meningococci should be given. Influenza vaccines are formulated each year based on predictions of the types of influenza viruses that will be circulating.[17] The vaccine is recommended for children over the age of 6 months who have underlying cardiac disease. Two doses given 1 month apart are required

Table 1 Usual Immunization Schedule

Age	Vaccine
2 months	DTP[1]; OPV[2]
4 months	DTP; OPV
6 months	DTP
15 months	MMR[3]; DTP; OPV
18 months	HIB[4]
4–6 years	DTP; OPV
14–16 years	Td[5]

[1]DTP = diphtheria and tetanus toxoids and pertussis vaccine adsorbed; [2]OPV = oral poliovirus vaccine (live); [3]MMR = measles, mumps and rubella virus vaccine (live); [4]HIB = *H. influenzae* type B conjugate vaccine; [5]Td = tetanus and diphtheria toxoids adsorbed (for adult use).

Table 2 Immunization Schedule for Older Children

Child is Under 7 Years of Age	
First visit	DTP[1]; OPV[2]; MMR[3]; HIB[4]
2 months later	DTP; OPV
2 months later	DTP
6–10 months later	DTP; OPV
Age 4–6 years	DTP; OPV
Age 14–16 years	Td[5]
Child is Over 7 Years of Age	
First visit	Td; OPV, MMR
2 months later	Td; OPV
6–12 months later	Td; OPV
Age 14–16 years	Td

[1]DTP = diphtheria and tetanus toxoids and pertussis vaccine adsorbed; [2]OPV = oral poliovirus vaccine (live); [3]MMR = measles, mumps and rubella virus vaccine (live); [4]HIB = *H. influenzae* type B conjugate vaccine; [5]Td = tetanus and diphtheria toxoids adsorbed (for adult use).

initially. The whole-cell vaccine is somewhat more immunogenic, but reactions to this vaccine are more frequent than with the split-virus product. The preferred vaccine for children is the split-virus formulation.[18] The vaccine should be given in the fall. Yearly vaccination is required because the types of viruses that circulate vary and immunity is imperfect. After the first season, a single immunization is adequate. Pneumococcal vaccine is effective in decreasing the incidence of pneumococcal infection.[19] Children with congenital heart disease are at higher risk for severe infection due to this agent. Furthermore, if polysplenia or aspenia is present, the risk for infection with pneumococci and other encapsulated organisms is greatly increased.[20] Pneumococcal vaccine is safe and immunogenic in children 2 years of age or older.[21] The vaccine consists of antigen from multiple (14 to 23) serotypes of *Streptococcus pneumoniae;* not all strains are immunogenic even in the 2-year-old child. The duration of immunity following vaccination is unclear. To date, booster immunizations have not been recommended. In adults who were revaccinated, there was an increase in local and systemic reactions.[22] It seems reasonable to vaccinate all children over the age of 2 years with serious heart disease. Consideration should be given to the use of meningococcal vaccine. Although there is no increase risk of infection reported in children with congenital heart disease, the vaccine is safe and effective. During immunosuppression, these patients will not reliably develop new antibodies. Thus, they will not become immune by carriage of the organism or by development of cross-reacting antibodies. For these reasons, it makes sense to protect the child by vaccination prior to transplantation.

A live, attenuated varicella vaccine has been extensively tested in the United States.[23,24] The vaccine is immunogenic, efficacious, and safe in both immunocompromised children and normal children. As soon as this vaccine is approved for use, it should be given to all transplant candidates who are susceptible to varicella. There are several studies that have documented safety, immunogenicity, and efficacy in children receiving chemotherapy for cancer; in most trials, immunosuppressive chemotherapy was discontinued for several weeks after vaccination.[25] In one trial, chemotherapy was continued and the vaccine was shown to be effective. In this trial, skin lesions due to vaccine virus occurred in most children; the illness was mild and self-limited in all but one child.[26] It is possible that vaccination of children receiving cyclosporine will be safe and efficacious. No data are available at this time.

Children with severe heart disease often require hospitalization. The major methods for preventing hospital-acquired infections are handwashing, isolation of infected patients, strict adherence to sterile technique, and minimizing the use of catheters and antibiotics.[27] Elective hospital admissions should be avoided during community outbreaks of influenza, respiratory syncytial virus, or other viruses because these agents are major nosocomial pathogens.[28] Isolation of infected children decreases the risk for nosocomial viral infection.[29]

Handwashing is essential for infection control.[30] Unfortunately, most physicians and many nurses neglect this simple procedure. In a study of handwashing frequency prior to and after contact with children hospitalized in an intensive care unit, Donowitz reported that physicians washed their hands in only 21% of contacts and nurses in only 47% of contacts.[31] Lack of handwashing will negate almost all other infection-control measures.

The use of indwelling catheters greatly increases the risk for nosocomial infection.[32] Catheters should be used only as medically necessary; the catheter should be removed as soon as possible.[33] Catheters in peripheral veins should be removed after 72 hours. Studies have clearly demonstrated that the risk for catheter-related bacteremia and sepsis rises dramatically after the catheter has been in place for 3 days.[34] Establishing protocols for catheter care and use of a "I.V. team" diminish the incidence of catheter-related infection.[35] Catheters placed into large central vessels often remain in place for long periods. The use of these central lines should be minimized. Tunneling the catheter below the skin and use of a Dacron cuff on the catheter serve to anchor the tube and thus decrease the movement of the catheter across the colonized skin of the insertion site and into the subcutaneous tissues. Infection rates for these indwelling, tunneled catheters range from 0.1 to 0.68 infections per 100 catheter days.[36] Infection rates are higher with double- or triple-lumen catheters.[37] Infection of indwelling catheters occurs when organisms ascend from the skin insertion site along the tunnel and into the vessel or when organisms enter the tubing via stopcocks, transducers, or drip chambers. Aseptic technique is essential whenever the catheter tubing is entered. Certain skin organisms, i.e., coagulase-negative staphylococci, especially *S. epidermidis,* have the ability to produce slime. This slime offers an adherence advantage; in addition, slime covers the organism, protecting it from host defenses.[38] Scanning catheters by electron microscopy reveals that most indwelling catheters are colonized by gram-positive cocci.[39] A variety of catheter dressings are in use; studies show no difference in infection rates with the use of transparent or gauze dressings.[40] Occlusive dressings are harmful because the skin under the dressing becomes macerated and damaged by the increased moisture, and damaged skin is more likely to become colonized by bacterial pathogens. Central catheters, which are placed percutaneously without use of a skin tunnel, are at the same or higher risk for infection as peripheral catheters. Increased manipulation of the catheter and breaks in sterile technique increase the rate of catheter-related infection. The use of stopcocks increases the risk of contamination of fluids infused via the catheters. Ports on the stopcocks are often left uncovered and sterile technique is often overlooked when samples are obtained or drugs infused.[41] Changing catheters over a wire has become standard practice. There is no evidence that this decreases the rate of infection. If the skin site is not properly disinfected, the risk for infection actually increases. Antibiotic therapy does not prevent or decrease the incidence of catheter-related infection. Rather, the use of antibiotics selects for colonization by resistant flora. Venous and arterial catheters increase a child's risk for nosocomial infection. The risks and benefits of catheter use must be taken into account in management decisions. Swan-Ganz catheters pose an even greater risk; these catheters cross and damage the heart valves. Autopsy studies show valvular damage and vegetations in over 50% of patients with indwelling Swan-Ganz catheters.[42] A damaged valve is at greater risk of becoming infected and causing endocarditis.

Catheters are often placed into the urinary bladder. Foley catheters place the child at risk for bacteruria and urinary tract infection. Studies have proven that the drainage system must be closed.[43] Sterile technique should be used whenever the system is entered, i.e., for drainage or to obtain samples of urine for laboratory studies.[44] Meatal-care regimens have been studied.[45] Incidence of bacteruria was compared in patients who had a variety of methods of perineal care; no care, cleansing with green soap, or cleasing with, and the application of, povidone-iodine solution and ointment. Surprisingly, no care resulted in the lowest rate of infection. In this study, manipulation of the catheter during cleasing of the skin increased the risk for infection. It is likely that manipulation of venous catheters during dressing changes increases the risk for bacteremia. In summary, catheters should be used for the shortest time possible; aseptic technique is critical and manipulation of the entrance site of the catheter should be minimized.

Peritransplantation

Infections immediately following transplantation are similar to those following any major surgery.[46,47] Atelectasis predisposes to bacterial pneumonia. Mechanical ventilation bypasses normal upper airway defenses. Morphine and other analgesics inhibit normal functioning of pulmonary macrophages. High concentrations of oxygen and high pressures damage cilia.[8] Wound infections, sternal osteomyelitis, and mediastinitis complicate open heart surgery.[48] Catheter-related infections include bacteruria and bacteremia (see Pretransplantation).

It is often difficult to distinguish septicemia from multiple-organ failure and infectious pneumonia from pulmonary edema. In fact, infection and failure often coexist. Antibiotic therapy should be limited as much as possible. Although antibiotic prophylaxis is uniformly given, the benefit in open heart surgery has not been proven. When antibiotics are used prophylactically, the duration of therapy should be limited. The first dose is given 1/2 hour prior to skin incision; subsequent doses are given for no longer than 48 hours.[49] Continuing antibiotics until drains and catheters are removed does not prevent infection and increases the risk for colonization or infection with resistant pathogens.

The benefit of protective isolation has not been proven for heart transplant recipients. Studies in bone-marrow transplantation patients and in children with leukemia show that protective isolation has no effect on survival.[50] The practice is inconvenient and expensive, especially if sterile gowns and gloves are required.[51] It is not surprising that protective isolation fails to prevent infections because most infections arise from the patient's endogenous flora.

Posttransplantation

The amount of morbidity due to infection is directly related to the extent of immunosuppression required to prevent graft rejection.[5–8] Cyclosporine acts selectively on T helper cells; the drug inhibits the production of growth factors needed for the normal function of B cells and cytotoxic T cells.[52] Cyclosporine impairs the production of interleukin-2 by T cells. These same T cells are necessary for normal cellular immunity, for antigen processing, and for modulation of humoral immunity. Patients with T-cell dysfunction are at increased risk for infection with usual, as well as opportunistic, pathogens.

Pathogens that require cell-mediated immunity for control include intracellular bacteria (e.g., *Salmonella, Listeria, Mycobacteria*), viruses, parasites, and fungi. Infections with opportunistic agents occur most commonly during and after the second month following transplantation. Bacteria cause a variety of illnesses. *Listeria monocytogenes,* a gram-positive bacillus, causes meningitis and septicemia. *Salmonella* species cause gastroenteritis; bacteremia often accompanies gastrointestinal disease. Joints, bones, soft tissues, and organs are involved as extraintestinal foci of *Salmonella*. *Legionella* is a major cause of pneumonia in adults following heart transplantation.[53] The organism has occasionally caused similar illness in compromised children.[54] Both typical and atypical mycobacteria cause pneumonia and disseminated disease in compromised hosts. The antibiotic susceptibilities of atypical mycobacteria are unpredictable. Diagnosis of mycobacterial infection is difficult. Skin tests are not reliable in these patients. Furthermore, granuloma formation does not always occur; a high index of suspicion is needed. Specific culture media and special stains are used to isolate and identify acid-fast bacteria.

Members of the herpes virus family cause significant morbidity in transplant recipients.[55] All members of this group cause latent infection. Primary infection and illness due to reactivation occur. Viruses in this family include herpes simplex (HSV), varicella-zoster (VZV), Epstein-Barr (EBV), and cytomegalovirus (CMV).

Herpes simplex virus type 1 is the cause of gingivostomatitis, recurrent "cold sores," esophagitis, and encephalitis. In the compromised host, HSV 1 recurs frequently. Local recurrence is usually just an annoyance, whereas pulmonary or gastrointestional infections cause significant morbidity.

Diagnosis depends on virus isolation or histologic study. Therapy is available and effective. Acyclovir shortens viral shedding and speeds healing; given daily, acyclovir prevents reactivation of the virus.[56,57] As with many drugs, there are interactions between cyclosporine and acyclovir. Thus, the risk of prophylaxis often outweighs the benefits of preventing recurrent HSV type 1 infections. HSV type 2 is the cause of genital ulcers; it has not yet been associated with excess morbidity in transplant recipients. It seems likely that in this population, recurrence rates with type 2 virus will be similar to those of type 1.

Varicella-zoster virus causes both chicken pox and shingles. The virus remains latent in ganglion cells following primary infection. Varicella is especially severe in compromised hosts; mortality rates of 7% are reported in untreated children with leukemia.[58] Early therapy with acyclovir shortens the course of the illness.[59] Zoster occurs more frequently in compromized hosts; further, the virus may disseminate to other skin dermatomes or to multiple organs. Therapy decreases the duration of symptoms and prevents dissemination.[60]

Epstein-Barr virus has been associated with Burkitt's lymphoma and nasopharyngeal carcinoma.[61] In organ transplant recipients, lymphomas of the central nervous system have occurred; EBV viral DNA has been identified in the tumor cells.[62,63] Currently, there is no known effective therapy for EBV.

Cytomegalovirus (CMV) is a major cause of morbidity after the first posttransplantation month.[64–68] The virus causes asymptomatic viruria, fever, a mononucleosis-like syndrome, pneumonitis, myocarditits, hepatitis, retinitis, and graft dysfunction. Primary infection follows an incubation period of 4 to 6 weeks and is associated with more severe illness. The usual source of infection is the transplanted organ or transfused blood.[67,69,70] There is clear evidence that primary disease follows transplantation of seropositive organs into seronegative recipients. The illness can be modified by the infusion of antibody to CMV. In renal transplant recipients, the incidence of illness due to CMV decreased from 60% to 20% in patients who received intravenous gammaglobulin.[71] Viral shedding was not different. Thus, immunoglobulin does not prevent infection, but modifies the illness, preventing symptoms and organ dysfunction. A new antiviral agent, gancyclovir has some efficacy in treatment of infections due to CMV.[72,73] The drug is not yet approved for use in children. Studies have shown improvement in symptoms and survival in patients with retinitis, gastrointestinal infection, and pneumonia. An attenuated CMV vaccine was developed and tested in seronegative recipients of renal transplants from seropositive donors.[74] Although vaccination prevented illness, it did not prevent infection. At this time, the vaccine is not available and has not been approved for use.

Influenza and respiratory syncytial virus (RSV) cause severe infection in children with underlying heart or lung disease.[75,76] It is likely that illness in transplant recipients will often be severe.[77] Pneumonia and bronchiolitis follow infection. Fever is variable during infections with RSV, but is a hallmark of influenza. Diagnosis is confirmed by recovery of the virus or detection of viral antigen in nasal wash specimens. Ribavirin given by aerosol prevents progression of disease and shortens the duration of symptoms.[78] Influenza vaccine should be given yearly. There is little information regarding antibody response in patients receiving cyclosporine. Immunization is not contraindicated because this is not a live vaccine.

Organ transplant recipients are at risk for infection with *Pneumocystis carinii*.[79,80] This agent is acquired early in life; immunosuppression leads to reactivation and the development of pneumonia.[81] The classic presenting symptoms are fever and respiratory distress. Physical findings are limited to the respiratory tract; retractions and dyspnea are severe, but rales are absent. Hypoxemia is universal. Radiographic findings include underaeration due to poor lung compliance and diffuse interstitial infiltrates with perihilar, peribronchial thickening. Diagnosis is established by histologic examination of bronchial alveolar lavage specimens or lung biopsy. The organism is stained by silver dyes. Both trimethoprim–sulfamethoxazole and pentamidine are effective therapy.[82] Unfortunately, dual infection with CMV, other viruses, and bacteria occur and respond poorly to therapy. Trimethoprim–sulfamethoxazole given three times a week prevents *P. carinii* infection in children with leukemia.[83] The risk of drug interaction and toxicity must be weighed against the benefit of prevention of *P. carinii* infection in transplant recipients. Use of prophylaxis should be based on the incidence of infection in each transplant center.

Toxoplasmosis has been reported to cause illness in the recipients of heart transplants.[84] A variety of illnesses follow primary infection: a mononucleosis-like syndrome, retinitis, encephalitis, myocarditis, and pneumonia. Reactivation of toxoplasmosis following cardiac transplantation is frequent and usually asymptomatic. Diagnosis depends on detection of antibody or demonstration of the parasite in biopsy specimens. Pyrimethamine–sulfadiazine therapy is effective against actively replicating organisms, but does not destroy encysted organisms.

Fungal infections occur most often as superinfections.[4–6] The risk for fungal infection is greatest in patients receiving multiple antibiotics, hyperalimentation, and in those with indwelling catheters. Candidiasis, aspergillosis, and mucomycosis are all reported in recipients of organ transplants. Early therapy with amphotericin B is needed to control the infection. Both *Aspergillus* and *Mucor* invade blood vessels and cause thrombosis; resection of this infarcted tissue is often required. A high index of suspicion and aggressive diagnostic studies are often needed to diagnose fungal infection prior to autopsy.

One of the most frequent sites of infection in patients with cardiac transplants is the lung.[4,85] Infections occur due to usual bacteria and viruses or due to any of the agents discussed in this section. Furthermore, pulmonary infiltrates result from noninfectious causes, such as pulmonary edema, emboli, and drug reactions.[86,87] Infections are often mixed. It appears that infection with cytomegalovirus predisposes to superinfection by bacteria, fungi, or *P. carinii*.[88] Infection in the lungs often progresses rapidly, resulting in respiratory failure and death.[89] For this reason, it is essential to establish a diagnosis and initiate appropriate therapy promptly. Evaluation of the patient with respiratory complaints begins with a complete history of the illness, a detailed physical examination, a chest radiograph, blood gas determination, and determination of the blood counts. Findings are often nonspecific. If the illness is progressing or hypoxemia is present, additional diagnostic studies are necessary. Cultures of blood and sputum for viruses, bacteria, and fungi should be obtained. Bronchoalveolar lavage (BAL) has become the diagnostic study of choice in children, as well as in adults.[90–94] The specimen is sent for histologic study and culture. The diagnostic sensitivity of BAL is quite high for *P. carinii*, viruses, and fungi. Quantitative cultures of BAL fluid are used to determine the role of bacteria.[95] If after completion of BAL no diagnosis is established, an open lung biopsy must be considered.[96,97] Empiric therapy should include antibiotics with activity against gram-positive and gram-negative bacteria and trimethoprim–sulfamethoxazole for *P. carinii*. Antivirals, such as ribavirin for suspected RSV, acyclovir for HSV, or ganciclovir for CMV, should be considered. In some cases, antifungal agents will also be necessary. Because of the multitude of therapeutic agents, the toxicities of these drugs, their interactions, and the intravenous fluids needed for delivery of the multiple agents, it is essential to establish a diagnosis and limit therapy. The outcome of pulmonary infection depends on the infecting agent, the state of the host, and the adequacy of therapy.

Summary

Infections cause significant morbidity and mortality in children with end-stage heart disease and in those who have undergone transplantation. Several illnesses can be prevented by immunizing the child prior to immunosuppression. Each child should receive the usual immunization (Table 1). In addition, influenza vaccine should be administered yearly, and pneumococcal and meningococcal vaccines should be given once after age 2 years. Elective admissions during viral outbreaks should be avoided. The best method to prevent nosocomial infection is handwashing. Every person who has contact with the patient must wash their hand prior to, and after, that contact. Sterile technique is mandatory during invasive procedures and during any manipulation of a catheter. The use of catheters and antibiotics should be minimized. Aggressive diagnosis and therapy of opportunistic infections will decrease morbidity and mortality. The benefits of antibiotic prophylaxis must be weighed against the risks of drug interaction and toxicity.

References

1. Stinson EB, Bieber CP, Griepp RB, et al: Infectious complications after cardiac transplantation in man. Ann Intern Med 1971, 74:22.
2. Addonizio LJ, Rose EA: Cardiac transplantation in children and adolescents. J Pediatr 1987, 111:1034.

3. Fricker FJ, Griffith BP, Hardesty RL, et al: Experience with heart transplantation in children. Pediatrics 1987, 79:138.
4. Ho M, Wajszczuk CP, Hardy A, et al: Infections in kidney, heart, and liver transplant recipients on cyclosporine. Transplant Proc 1983, 15:2768.
5. Mason JW, Stinson EB, Hunt SA, et al: Infections after cardiac transplantation: Relation to rejection therapy. Ann Inten Med 1976, 85:69.
6. Hofflin JM, Potasman I, Baldwin JC, et al: Infectious complications in heart transplant recipients receiving cyclosporine and corticosteroids. Ann Intern Med 1987, 106:209.
7. Rubin RH, Wolfson JS, Cosimi AB, et al: Infection in the renal transplant recipient. Am J Med 1981, 70:405.
8. Oh C-S, Stratta RJ, Fox BC, et al: Increased infections associated with the use of OKT3 for treatment of steroid-resistant rejection in renal transplantation. Transplantation 1988, 45:68.
9. Fisher MC: Nosocomial pulmonary infections in children. J Thorac Imag 1986, 1:25.
10. Santos JI, Arredondo JL, Vitale JJ: Nutrition, infection and immunity. Pediatr Ann 1983, 12:182.
11. Katz MK, Stiehm ER: Host defense in malnutrition. Pediatrics 1977, 59: 490.
12. Johanson WG, Pierce AK, Sanford JP: Changing pharyngeal bacterial flora of hospitalized patients Emergence of gram-negative bacilli. N Engl J Med 1969, 281:137.
13. Harris AA, Levin S, Trenholme GM: Selected aspects of nosocomial infections in the 1980s. Am J Med 1984, 77(Suppl):3.
14. Ginsburg CM, Andrews A: Orthotopic hepatic transplantation for unimmunized children: A paradox of contemporary medical care. Pediatr Infect Dis J 1987, 6:764.
15. Fulginite VA: Incomplete immunizations, hospitalization, and specialty care. An opportunity to improve the immunization status of very young children. (Editorial) Am J Dis Child 1988, 142:704.
16. Campbell AGM: Immunisation for the immunosuppressed child. Arch Dis Child 1988, 63:113.
17. Immunization Practices Advisory Committee. Prevention and control of influenza. MMWR 1988, 37:361.
18. Hall CB: Influenza: A shot or not? Pediatrics 1987, 79:564.
19. Giebink GS: Preventing pneumococcal disease in children: Recommendations for using pneumococcal vaccine. Pediatr Infect Dis 1985, 4:343.
20. Waldman JD, Rosenthal A, Smith AL, et al: Sepsis and congenital asplenia. J Pediatr 1977, 90:555.
21. Lawrence EM, Edwards KM, Schiffman G, et al: Pneumococcal vaccine in normal children. Primary and secondary vaccination. Am J Dis Child 1983, 137:846.
22. Schwartz JS: Pneumococcal vaccine: Clinical efficacy and effectiveness. Ann Intern Med 1982, 96:208.
23. Weibel RE, Neff BJ, Kuter BJ, et al: Live attenuated varicella virus vaccine. Efficacy trial in healthy children. N Engl J Med 1984, 310:1409.

24. Johnson CE, Shurin PA, Fattlar D, et al: Live attenuated varicella vaccine in healthy 12- to 24-month-old children. Pediatrics 1988, 81:512.
25. Gershon AA, Steinberg SP, Gelb L, et al: Live attenuated varicella vaccine. Efficacy for children with leukemia in remission. JAMA 1984, 252:355.
26. Ha K, Baba K, Ikeda T, et al: Application of live varicella vaccine to children with acute leukemia or other malignancies without suspension of anticancer therapy. Pediatrics 1980, 65:346.
27. American Hospital Association. Infection Control in the Hospital. Revised edition. American Hospital Association Chicago, 1970.
28. Hall CB: Nosocomial viral respiratory infections: Perennial weeds on pediatric wards. Am J Med 1981, 70:670.
29. Valenti WM, Betts RF, Hall CB, et al: Nosocomial viral infections: II. Guidelines for prevention and control of respiratory viruses, herpesviruses, and hepatitis viruses. Infect Control 1980, 1:165.
30. Steere AC, Mallison GF: Handwashing practices for the prevention of nosocomial infections. Ann Intern Med 1975, 83:683.
31. Donowitz LG: Handwashing technique in pediatric intensive care unit. Am J Dis Child 1987, 141:683.
32. Maki DG: Nosocomial bacteremia. An epidemiologic overview. Am J Med 1981, 70:719.
33. Simmons BP: Guidelines for prevention of intravascular infections. In: Centers for Disease Control: Guidelines for the Prevention and Control of Nosocomial Infections. Public Health Service, Atlanta; 1981, pp. 61–71.
34. Maki DG, Boldmnan DA, Rhame FS: Infection control in intravenous therapy. Ann Intern Med 1973, 79:867.
35. Tomford JW, Hershey CO, McLaren CE, et al: Intravenous therapy and peripheral venous catheter-associated complications. A prospective controlled study. Arch Intern Med 1984, 144:1191.
36. Wurzel CL, Halom K, Feldman JG, et al: Infection rates of Broviac-Hickman catheters and implantable venous devices. Am J Dis Child 1988, 142:536.
37. Hilton E, Haslett TM, Borenstein MT, et al: Central catheter infections: Single- versus triple-lumen catheters. Influence of guide wires on infection rates when used for replacement of catheters. Am J Med 1988, 84: 667.
38. Quie PG, Belani KK: Coagulase-negative staphylococcal adherence and persistence. J Infect Dis 1987, 156:543.
39. Marrie TJ, Costerton JW: Scanning and transmission electron microscopy of in situ bacterial colonization and intraarterial catheters. J Clin Micro 1984, 19:687.
40. Maki DG, Ringer M: Evaluation of dressing regimens for prevention of infection with peripheral intravenous catheters. Gauze, a transparent polyurethane dressing, and an iodophor-transparent dressing. JAMA 1987, 258:2396.
41. Brosnan KM, Parham AM, Rutledge B, et al: Stopcock. Am J Nursing 1988, 88:320.
42. Rowley KM, Clubb KS, Smith GJW, et al: Right-sided infective endocardi-

tis as a consequence of flow-directed pulmonary-artery catheterization. A clinicopathological study of 55 autopsied patients. N Engl J Med 1984, 311:1152.
43. Garibaldi RA, Burke JP, Dickman ML, et al: Factors predisposing to bacteriuria during indwelling urethral catheterization. N Engl J Med 1974, 291:215.
44. Stamm WE: Guidelines for prevention of catheter-associated urinary tract infections. Ann Intern Med 1975, 82:386.
45. Burke JP, Garibaldi RA, Britt MR, et al: Prevention of catheter-associated urinary tract infections. Efficacy of daily meatal care regimens. Am J Med 1981, 70:655.
46. Altemeier WA: Surgical infections: Incisional wounds. In Bennett JV, Brachman PS, eds: Hospital Infections. Boston: Brown and Co., Little, 1979, pp. 287–306.
47. Stone HH: Infection in postoperative patients. Am J Med 1988, 81(Suppl IA):39.
48. Firmin RK, Wood A: Postoperative sternal wound infections. Infect Surg 1987, 6:231.
49. Kesler RW, Guhlow LJ, Saulsbury FT: Prophylactic antibiotics in pediatric surgery. Pediatrics 1982, 69:1.
50. Nauseef WM, Maki DG: A study of the value of simple protective isolation in patients with granulocytopenia. N Engl J Med 1981, 304:448.
51. Armstrong D: Protected environments are discomforting and expensive and do not offer meaningful protection. Am J Med 1984, 76:685.
52. Cohen DJ, Loertscher R, Rubin MF, et al: Cyclosporine: A new immunosuppressive agent for organ transplantation. Ann Intern Med 1984, 101:667.
53. Fuller J, Levinson MM, Kline JR, et al: Legionnaires' disease after heart transplantation. Ann Thorac Surg 1985, 39:308.
54. Ryan ME, Feldman S, Pruitt B, et al: Legionnaires' disease in a child with cancer. Pediatrics 1979, 64:951.
55. Pollard RB, Arvin AM, Gamberg P, et al: Specific cell-mediated immunity and infections with herpes viruses in cardiac transplant recipients. Am J Med 1982, 73:679.
56. Gold D, Corey L: Acyclovir prophylaxis for herpes simplex virus infection. Antimicrob Agents Chemother 1987, 31:361.
57. Chou S, Gallagher JG, Merigan TC: Controlled clinical trial of intravenous acyclovir in heart-transplant patients with mucocutaneous herpes simplex infections. Lancet 1981, i:1392.
58. Feldman S, Hughes WT, Daniel CB: Varicella in children with cancer: Seventy-seven cases. Pediatrics 1975, 56:388.
59. Nyerges G, Meszner Z, Gyarmati E, et al: Acyclovir prevents dissemination of varicella in immunocompromised children. J Infect Dis 1988, 157:309.
60. Balfour HH, Bean B, Laskin OL, et al: Acyclovir halts progression of herpes zoster in immunocompromised patients. N Engl J Med 1983, 308:1448.
61. Sullivan JL, Medveczky P, Forman SJ, et al: Epstein-Barr-virus induced

lymphoproliferation. Implications for antiviral chemotherapy. N Engl J Med 1984, 311:1163.
62. Dummer JS, Bound LM, Singh G, et al: Epstein-Barr-virus-induced lymphoma in a cardiac transplant recipient. Am J Med 1984, 77:179.
63. Hanto DW, Frizzera G, Gajl-Peczalska KJ, et al: Epstein-Barr virus-induced lymphoma after renal transplantation. Acyclovir therapy and transition from polyclonal to monoclonal B-cell proliferation. N Engl J Med 1982, 306:913.
64. Preiksaitis JK, Rosno S, Grumet C, et al: Infections due to herpesviruses in cardiac transplant recipients: Role of the donor heart and immunosuppressive therapy. J Infect Dis 1983, 147:974.
65. Dummer JS, White LT, Ho M, et al: Morbidity of cytomegalovirus infection in recipients of heart or heart-lung transplants who received cyclosporine. J Infect Dis 1985, 152:1182.
66. Chou S: Cytomegalovirus infection and reinfection transmitted by heart transplantation. J Infect Dis 1987, 155:1054.
67. Summer JS, Hardy A, Poorsattar A, et al: Early infections in kidney, heart, and liver-transplant recipients on cyclosporine. Transplantation 1983, 36: 259.
68. Preiksaitis JK, Brown L, McKenzie M: The risk of cytomegalovirus infection in seronegative transfusion recipients not receiving exogenous immunosuppression. J Infect Dis 1988, 157:523.
69. Gorensek MJ, Stewart RW, Keys TF, et al: A multivariate analysis of the risk of cytomegalovirus infection in heart transplant recipients. J Infect Dis 1988, 157:515.
70. Pass RF: Epidemiology and transmission of cytomegalovirus. J Infect Dis 1985, 152:243.
71. Snydman DR, Werner BG, Heinze-Lacey B, et al: Use of cytomegalovirus immune globulin to prevent cytomegalovirus disease in renal-transplant recipients. N Engl J Med 1987, 317:1049.
72. Collaborative DHPG Treatment Study Group. Treatment of serious cytomegalovirus infections with 9-(1,3-dihydroxy-2-propoxymethyl) guanine in patients with AIDS and other immunodeficiencies. N Engl J Med 1986, 314:801.
73. Harbison MA, DeGirolami PC, Jenkins RL, et al: Ganciclovir therapy of severe cytomegalovirus infections in solid-organ transplant recipients. Transplantation 1988, 46:82.
74. Piotkin SA, Smiley ML, Friedman HM, et al: Towne-vaccine-induced prevention of cytomegalovirus disease after renal transplants. Lancet 1984, i:528.
75. Cooper ER: The epidemiology of influenza in childhood. J Resp Dis 1987, 8(Suppl):s23.
76. MacDonald NE, Hall CB, Suffin SC, et al: Respiratory syncytial viral infection in infants with congenital heart disease. N Engl J Med 1982, 307:397.
77. Ogra PL, Patel J: Respiratory syncytial virus infection and the immunocompromised host. Pediatr Infect Dis J 1988, 7:246.

78. Hall CB, McBride JT, Gala CL, et al: Ribavirin treatment of respiratory syncytial viral infection in infants with underlying cardiopulmonary disease. JAMA 1985, 254:3047.
79. Gryzan S, Paradis IL, Zeevi A, et al: Unexpectedly high incidence of *Pneumocystis carinii* infection after lung-heart transplantation. Implications for lung defense and allograft survival. Am Rev Respir Dis 1988, 137:1268.
80. Hardy AM, Wajszczuk CP, Suffredini AF, et al: *Pneumocystis carinii* pneumonia in renal-transplant recipients treated with cyclosporine and steroids. J Infect Dis 1984, 149:143.
81. Hughes WT: *Pneumocystis carinii* pneumonia. N Engl J Med 1977, 297:1381.
82. Wharton JM, Coleman DL, Wofsy CB, et al: Trimethoprim–sulfamethoxazole or pentamidine for pneumocystis carinii pneumonia in the acquired immunodeficiency syndrome. A prospective randomized trial. Ann Intern Med 1986, 105:37.
83. Hughes WT, Rivera GK, Schell MJ, et al: Successful intermittent chemoprophylaxis for *Pneumocystis carinii* pneumonitis. N Engl J Med 1987, 316:1627.
84. Luft BJ, Naot Y, Araujo FG, et al: Primary and reactivated toxoplasma infection in patients with cardiac transplants. Clinical spectrum and problems in diagnosis in a defined population. Ann Intern Med 1983, 99:27.
85. Mammana RB, Petersen EA, Fuller JK, et al: Pulmonary infections in cardiac transplant patients: Modes of diagnosis, complications, and effectiveness of therapy. Ann Thor Surg 1983, 36:700.
86. Rosenow EC III, Wilson WR, Cockerill FR III: Pulmonary disease in the immunocompromised host (first of two parts). Mayo Clin Proc 1985, 60:473.
87. Wilson WR, Cockerill FR III, Rosenow EC III: Pulmonary disease in the immunocompromised host (second of two parts). Mayo Clin Proc 1985, 60:610.
88. Rand KH, Pollard RB, Merigan TC: Increased pulmonary superinfections in cardiac-transplant patients undergoing primary cytomegalovirus infection. N Engl J Med 1978, 298:951.
89. Masur H, Shelhamer J, Parrillo JE: The management of pneumonias in immunocompromised patients. JAMA 1985, 253:1769.
90. Reynolds HY: Bronchoalveolar lavage. Am Rev Respir Dis 1987, 135:250.
91. Stover DE, Zaman MB, Hajdu SI, et al: Bronchoalveolar lavage in the diagnosis of diffuse pulmonary infiltrates in the immunosuppressed host. Ann Intern Med 1984, 101:1.
92. Springmeyer SC, Hackman RC, Holle R, et al: Use of bronchoalveolar lavage to diagnose acute diffuse pneumonia in the immunocompromised host. J Infect Dis 1986, 154:604.
93. Frankel LR, Smith DW, Lewiston NJ: Bronchoalveolar lavage for diagnosis of pneumonia in the immunocompromised child. Pediatrics 1988, 81:785.
94. Pattishall EN, Noyes BE, Orenstein DM: Use of bronchoalveolar lavage in

immunocompromised children with pneumonia. Pediatr Pulmonol 1988, 5:1.
95. Kahn FW, Jones JM: Diagnosing bacterial respiratory infection by bronchoalveolar lavage. J Infect Dis 1987, 155:862.
96. Prober CG, Whyte H, Smith CR: Open lung biopsy in immunocompromised children with pulmonary infiltrates. Am J Dis Child 1984, 138:60.
97. Imoke E, Dudgeon DL, Colombani P, et al: Open lung biopsy in the immunocompromised pediatric patient. J Pediatr Surg 1983, 18:816.

Chapter 14

Postoperative Evaluation of Pediatric Transplant Patients

Richard M. Donner, Craig R. Cohen, and David A. Burton

Cardiac Mechanics

A description of the mechanical properties of the transplanted heart is essential if we are to evaluate the effects of donor–recipient size mismatching, the adaption of the heart to the normal growth process, and the effects of acute and chronic graft rejection. There are no systematic studies of cardiac mechanics in pediatric transplant recipients, partly because the number of patients in each center is small, and intermediate and late follow-up groups contain only a few subjects. Much of what is known is drawn from adult studies or combined studies that contain one or two children each. Although some similarity seems to exist between cardiac mechanics in the adult and child recipient, there is no guarantee that the populations will be identical.

It is most advantageous to describe cardiac mechanics in terms of three categories: hemodynamics, pump function (the ability of the heart to act as a pump), and contractile function (an assessment of the contractile ability of the myocardium). Emphasis is first placed on the resting state; a discussion of exercise hemodynamics and functional reserve follows in the next section.

Hemodynamics

Most adult and combined series report an elevated resting heart rate,[1–4] although a few have encountered rates not significantly different from normal.[5,6] The most widely proposed mechanism for the

From *Heart Transplantation in Children*, edited by Jeffrey M. Dunn, M.D. and Richard M. Donner, M.D.

elevated rates is the lack of parasympathetic innervation. There does not seem to be a progressive decrease in the heart rate with time, suggestive of reinnervation. Stroke volume and cardiac index, related to the body surface area of the recipient, are normal in most series after the first month,[1,4–7] but diminished in a few.[2] Pulmonary artery pressure and vascular resistance are increased,[2,6] but decrease during the first postoperative year.[8] Mean aortic pressure and systemic vascular resistance are elevated and do not diminish over time.[2,5–7] Right and left ventricular filling pressures are generally abnormal early, but are normal or mildly elevated after 1 year.[1,2,6–8] However, some occult restrictive disease may persist,[6] perhaps related to, or made worse by, the significant incidence of tricuspid valve regurgitation.[6,9]

Hemodynamic studies in a small series of eight children, ages 5 months to 19 years, who underwent combined catheterization and echocardiography 4 months to 2 years after transplant at our institution, are shown in Table 1. A group of age-matched, normal children was selected for comparison. Resting heart rate was elevated. Stroke volume index was slightly decreased, but not significantly so. Cardiac index, computed by echocardiography, was also normal, consistent with other data in children.[10] Mean pulmonary arterial pressure was higher in transplant patients and pulmonary vascular resistance (Fick method with an assumed oxygen consumption) was mildly elevated, but not significantly different. Right ventricular end-diastolic pressure was mildly elevated. Studies in children have also shown elevated aortic pressure and systemic vascular resistance.[10] Although the total number of patients is small, the hemodynamics found in children after recovery from surgery are very similar to those of the adult.

Table 1. Hemodynamics in Eight Children Four Months to Two Years After Transplantation

	Transplant Patients	Age Matched Normal Children	*p* Value
Heart rate (beats/min)	104 ± 12	86 ± 11	<.05
SVI (cc/m^2)	26 ± 6	36 ± 8	NS
CI (L/min/m^2)	2.9 ± .5	3.0 ± .6	NS
Mean PAP (mm Hg)	21 ± 5	15 ± 4	<.04
PVR (Woods units)	3.0 ± 1.0	2.7 ± .7	NS
RVEDP (mm Hg)	8 ± 2	4 ± 2	<.02

SVI = stroke volume index; CI = cardiac index; PAP = pulmonary artery pressure; PVR = pulmonary vascular resistance; RVEDP = right ventricular end-diastolic pressure.

Pump Function

In adult and combined series, left ventricular end-diastolic volume is diminished,[2,5] even when related to the body surface area of the donor.[11] End-systolic volume was greatly diminished in one study.[5] Ejection fraction is reported as elevated,[5] normal,[7] or decreased.[2,3] These conflicting findings result from differences of measurement technique, immunosuppression regimens, postoperative timing of the study, and wide variation of control populations. In no study, however, did there appear to be a relation between the number of successfully treated moderate rejection episodes and ejection fraction.

Findings in seven of our children were most similar to those of Borow et al.[5] and are summarized in Table 2. Left ventricular end-diastolic and end-systolic volume indexes were reduced, and ejection fraction was mildly elevated.

Table 2. Pump and Contractile Function in Eight Children Four Months to Two Years After Transplantation

	Transplant Patients	Age Matched Normal Children	*p* Value
LVEDVI (cc/m²)	39 ± 7	54 ± 13	<.03
LVESVI (cc/m²)	11 ± 2	18 ± 5	<.01
EF (%)	72 ± 3	66 ± 4	<.01
Mean Vcf (circum/sec)	1.9 ± .2	1.1 ± .2	<.001
LVMI (gm/m²)	70 ± 15	55 ± 12	<.05
ES stress (gm/cm²)	29 ± 5	55 ± 8	<.001

LVEDVI = left ventricular end-diastolic volume index; LVESVI = left ventricular end-systolic volume index; EF = ejection fraction; Vcf = velocity of circumferential fiber shortening; LVMI = left ventricular mass index; ES stress = end-systolic stress.

Contractile function

In combined series of adults and a few children, left ventricular mass is increased.[5,6] Borow et al.[5] found that this increased mass was responsible for diminished end-systolic wall stress and the elevated pump performance (fractional shortening, ejection fraction) they observed. Further, this relationship between end-systolic stress and shortening was altered with infusion of dobutamine. A greater degree of shortening observed for a given end-systolic stress suggested that contractile reserve is present in the transplanted heart.

Similar findings were present in our children (Table 2). Left ventricular mass is greater and end-systolic stress is less in the transplant patients than in normals. Figure 1 shows the naturally occurring values of end-systolic stress in the transplant patients and in nine normal children. The inverse relationship between end-systolic stress and shortening (mean velocity of circumferential fiber shortening) is similar in both groups, suggesting that contractile function in transplant patients is normal, but increased left ventricular mass and diminished wall stress produce increased shortening.

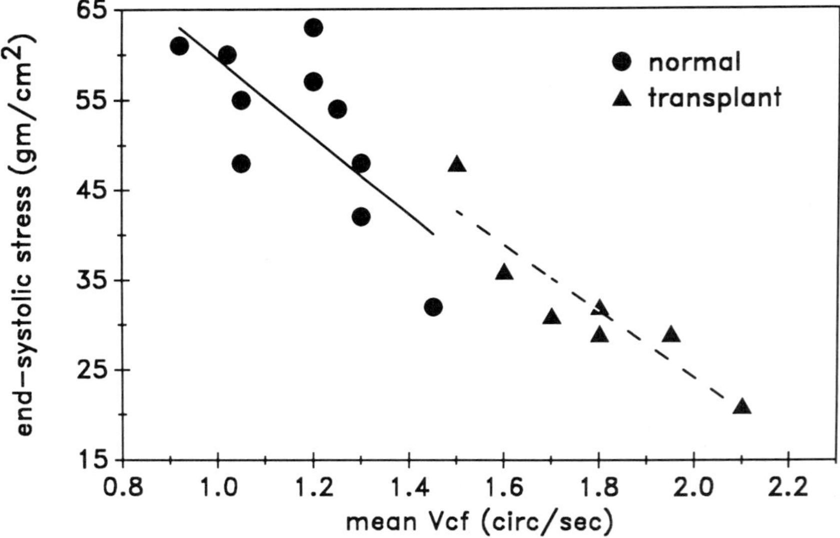

Figure 1: *The end-systolic, meridional, stress-shortening relationship in nine normal children and seven transplant patients. Simultaneous echocardiography and left ventricular pressure measurements were used to obtain stress and mean velocity of circumferential fiber shortening (Vcf).*

Exercise Evaluation

Cardiac hemodynamics at rest and during exercise are normally influenced by sympathetic and parasympathetic tone. In humans, reinnervation following transplantation does not occur.[12] The absence of these neural connections directly influences the cardiac transplant patient's response to exercise.

Exercise data in pediatric transplant recipients are scarce and often presented in mixed populations of adults and children. Exercise responses in adults are summarized in Table 3. During early exercise, cardiac hemodynamics are mostly influenced by increased systemic venous return from the exercising skeletal muscles. According to the Frank-Starling mechanism, there is an increase in end-diastolic volumes and pressures, resulting in an increased stroke volume.[13] Oxygen consumption is lower than expected, and there is a compensatory increase in tissue oxygen extraction (A-V oxygen difference).[1] There is a modest rise in the heart rate, which may be related to right atrial stretch mechanisms that are not fully understood.[14] The plasma norepinephrine levels are not yet significantly increased. In mid and late exercise, the increase in cardiac performance is a consequence of increased circulating catecholamines. The increase in circulating norepinephrine causes a dramatic increase in heart rate and cardiac output, although end-diastolic, end-systolic, and stroke volumes are decreased.[13,15] Oxygen consumption remains low in relation to cardiac output and the A-V oxygen difference widens further. At peak exercise, blood lactate levels are higher than normal; this is reflected in an elevated anaerobic threshold. The total work performed is usually less than normal.[1,13] In summary, the major difference in the exercise response between a normally innervated heart and a denervated heart is the means by which they achieve their maximal response. In a native heart, at the onset of exercise, increased cardiac output results from a simultaneous increase in both stroke volume and heart rate from direct sympathetic stimulation. In the denervated heart, the early

Table 3. Exercise Responses in Adults

	Rest	Early-Mid Exercise	Peak Exercise
Heart rate	+	+	+ +
LVEDP	+/0	+ +	−
Stroke volume	−	+ +	+
Cardiac output	−/0	+ +	+ +
Oxygen consumption	− −	+	+
A-V oxygen difference	+	+ +	+ +
Plasma norepinephrine	0	+ +	+ + +
Blood lactate	0	+	+
Blood pressure	0	+ +	+ +

LVEDP = left ventricular end-diastolic pressure; 0 = normal resting value; +, + +, + + + = mild, moderate, great increase above normal resting value; −, − − = mild, moderate decrease below normal resting value.

increase in cardiac output is due to increased stroke volume from augmented systemic venous return. It is not until mid exercise, when circulating norepinephrine increases, that heart rate contributes to a further increase in cardiac output.

In our institution, five adolescents and young adults (four males and one female) underwent exercise stress testing after cardiac transplantation. Four patients had preexisting cardiomyopathy, and one had severe heart failure following mitral valve replacement for Marfan syndrome. At the time of stress testing, none had any significant arrhythmias or rejection by endomyocardial biopsy. All were maintained on an immunosuppressive regimen of cyclosporine, prednisone, and azathioprine, and two received antihypertensive therapy. All subjects were exercised to maximal voluntary exertion on a motorized treadmill using the Bruce protocol. Breath-by-breath collection of respiratory gasses were measured by mass spectrometry, and cardiac output was determined using the acetylene-helium rebreathing method. The results of these tests were compared to those of normal subjects matched according to body surface area.

The results of stress testing are summarized in Table 4. With the exception of heart rate, none of the resting values for transplant patients are significantly different from the normal group. However, the transplant patients had slightly higher cardiac outputs than did the control group, and the 0_2 pulse and stroke volume were slightly lower. With exercise, the transplant patients demonstrated a more gradual rate of rise to a lower peak heart rate than that of the controls (Fig. 2). At maximal exercise, there were also no significant differences between transplant patients and normals. Total work performed (METS) was slightly, but not significantly, less in transplant patients, and both groups stopped exercising for similar reasons, exhaustion or leg fatigue. Results of exercise electrocardiograms were unremarkable. None of the transplant patients or controls exhibited arrhythmias or significant ST–T wave changes. Five- minute recovery electrocardiograms were also normal for both groups.

Our transplant patients demonstrated a significantly elevated resting heart rate when compared to the normal children. This is consistent with observations in adults, but the resting heart rates for our younger transplant patients were higher than those generally seen in the adult transplant population. Although the increase in heart rate was slow during the early stages of exercise, it was more marked than that seen in a similar adult transplant group. It is difficult to draw

Table 4. Exercise Stress Testing in Five Teenagers and Young Adults

	Transplant Patients	Normal Children
Age at transplant (yrs)	17.6 ± 2.9	–
Age at stress testing (yrs)	18.4 ± 2.5	15.6 ± 1.2
Weight (kg)	77.2 ± 32.5	66.8 ± 14.3
BSA (m^2)	1.75 ± .34	1.70 ± .23
HR at rest (beats/min)	112 ± 12	85 ± 9
HR at maximal exercise (beats/min)	177 ± 10	186 ± 15
CI at rest ($l/min/m^2$)	3.03 ± 0.8	2.76 ± 0.9
CI at maximal exercise ($l/min/m^2$)	6.5 ± 1.2	6.6 ± 1.8
SVI at rest (cc/m^2)	27 ± 7	33 ± 6
SVI at maximal exercise (cc/m^2)	37 ± 9	36 ± 7
VO_2 at rest ($l/min/m^2$)	0.15 ± .06	0.16 ± .04
VO_2 at maximal exercise ($l/min/m^2$)	1.02 ± .40	1.25 ± .24
O_2 pulse at rest (cc/beat)	2.35 ± 0.83	3.03 ± 0.93
O_2 pulse at max exercise (cc/beat)	12.32 ± 4.89	11.32 ± 1.69
Ventilation at rest (l/min)	10.0 ± 4.1	9.4 ± 2.4
Ventilation at max exercise (l/min)	73.9 ± 28.3	59.4 ± 17.2
METS	12.12 ± .91	12.74 ± 1.71

HR = heart rate; CI = cardiac index; SVI = stroke volume index; VO_2 = oxygen consumption.

conclusions from this very small group of patients, but the mildly decreased level of work achieved (METS) by the transplant group suggests abnormal exercise physiology. The mildly diminished VO_2, stroke volume, and heart rate at maximal exercise might reflect the donor heart's inability to meet metabolic demands. The increased ventilatory rate and, possibly, a lower anaerobic threshold might be due to decreased oxygen delivery to the exercising muscles. The mild increase in O_2 pulse reflects increased oxygen extraction and could serve as a compensatory mechanism. Adult studies show a similar phenomenon: for any given VO_2, cardiac output is lower in transplant patients than in normals. It is unclear if the denervated state, inappropriate peripheral resistance, or other unknown factors are responsible for this finding.[1]

The results of the exercise stress tests in our patients must be interpreted with caution and serve only as a starting point in the in-

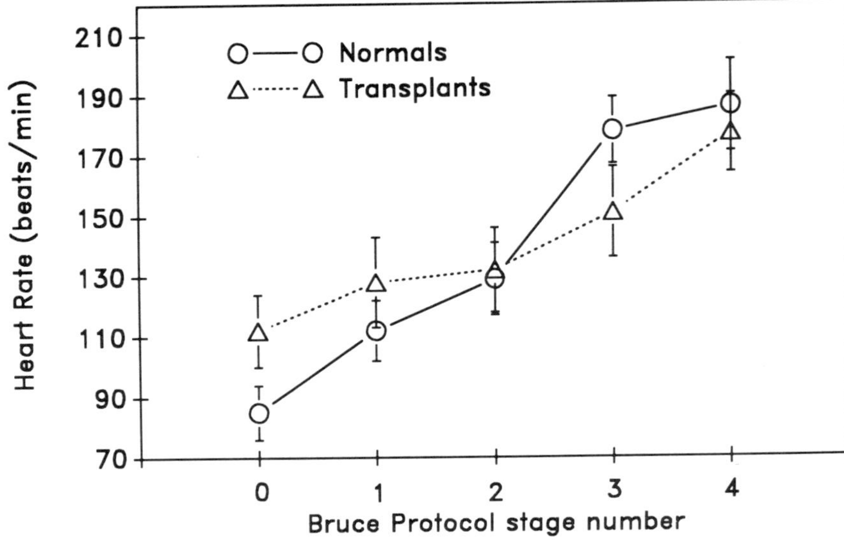

Figure 2: *Heart rate at Bruce protocol stages in transplant patients and normals. In transplant patients, heart rate is elevated at rest, but rises more slowly and is lower than normals at maximal exercise.*

vestigation of the functional capacity of the pediatric heart transplant patient. The many variables, such as age, donor–recipient size match, immunosuppression, and frequency and severity of acute and chronic rejection, that might affect this functional capacity will, of course, require a larger and more varied patient population.

Electrocardiography and Electrophysiology

Transplantation of the human heart provides a unique situation for studying the autonomic influences of the sympathetic and parasympathetic nervous systems on cardiac electrophysiologic function. The transplanted heart contains two sinus nodes. The donor sinus node lacks nervous innervation, and its function is therefore independent of nervous control. It is this sinus node that acts as the pacemaker of the heart. The recipient sinus node is also present because the technique of transplantation leaves the posterior portion of the heart in situ. This sinus node retains its normal nervous connections despite its electrical separation from the remainder of the donor heart. Thus, differential responses of the donor and recipient sinus nodes are explained by alterations in nervous control; these responses provide a model for studying autonomic influences on sinus node function.

Nervous Control of Electrophysiologic Function

The parasympathetic nervous system arises in the medulla of the brain and descends to form the vagus nerve. These preganglionic fibers synapse with postganglionic fibers located within the heart itself. Most of these cells are near the sinus and AV nodes. The right vagus predominantly affects the sinus node and stimulation of this nerve produces sinus bradycardia or cessation of electrical activity. The left vagus nerve affects the AV node to cause AV conduction delay. The fibers of the sympathetic nervous system originate in the spinal columns of the upper five or six thoracic and lower one or two cervical segments. These fibers enter the paravertebral chain of ganglia, synapse in the stellate ganglia or in the caudal cervical ganglia, and join the parasympathetic fibers to form a complex network to the heart. These fibers penetrate the heart with the coronary vessels and supply the SA node, the AV node, and the myocardium directly. The sympathetic receptors in the heart are beta receptors. The right-sided fibers predominantly affect heart rate, whereas the left sided fibers seem to affect contractility.

Reflexes controlling heart rate are numerous. The Bainbridge reflex is mediated through the vagus nerve. Receptors in the venoatrial junctions, such as the junctions of the right atrium with the vena cavae and the left atrium with the pulmonary veins, will cause acceleration of the heart rate with chamber distension. Baroreceptors, located in the aortic arch and carotid sinuses, respond to changes in blood pressure. Increased blood pressure suppresses the sympathetic system and augments vagus control, resulting in bradycardia. Reduced blood pressure augments the sympathetic system and suppresses the vagus, producing tachycardia. Respiratory sinus arrhythmia is mediated through the vagus nerve. Peripheral chemoreceptors and intrinsic autoregulation also affect heart rate. It is the combination of both direct nervous system responses, reflex control and autoregulation, that determines the heart rate at any point in time.

Resting heart rate is primarily under vagal control, which is dominant at the sinus node. Following transplantation, there is a removal of this resting parasympathetic tone, which results in a resting tachycardia. A regression formula to estimate the expected, intrinsic rate was determined in normal individuals by creating autonomic blockade with atropine and propranolol.[16–18]

$$\text{Intrinsic heart rate} = 117.2 - (0.53 \times \text{age})$$

The calculated intrinsic heart rate for any patient can be determined using this formula. A lower than calculated intrinsic heart rate may indicate sinus node dysfunction and will be discussed below.

Electrocardiography and Electrophysiologic Function

The 12-lead, resting electrocardiogram following transplantation usually demonstrates both donor and recipient P waves. The donor P waves are those associated with the QRS complex. The recipient P waves, usually at a slower rate, are unassociated with ventricular complexes and are usually more difficult to identify (Fig. 3). Atrial activity is always easily demonstrated during electrophysiologic study where

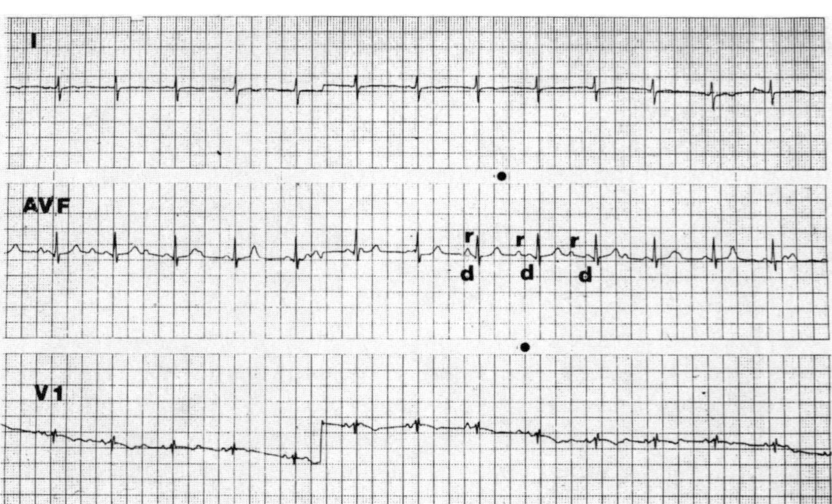

Figure 3: *Rhythm strip with three simultaneous leads (I, aV_F, V_1). Donor and recipient P waves are best seen in lead aV_F. Those labeled* d *are donor P waves and are associated with QRS complexes. Those labeled* r *are recipient P waves unassociated with QRS complexes.*

there is clear dissociation of donor and recipient atrial electrograms (Fig. 4).

Early sinus nodal dysfunction is common, and in this clinical setting, donor P waves may not be seen.[19] This dysfunction may be due to surgical trauma to the donor node or to its blood supply, prior abnormal sinus node dysfunction of the donor, prolonged ischemic time during procurement, or acute rejection. These abnormalities are usually transient and result in escape junctional rhythms. Of 10 pediatric patients in our series with early postoperative electrocardiograms, 5 had normal sinus rhythm, 4 had junctional rhythms, and 1 had a low atrial rhythm. All but one reverted to sinus rhythm prior to discharge. Early junctional rhythm (without donor P waves) with normal recipient P waves (unassociated with the QRS complexes) gives the electrocardiographic appearance of AV dissociation. This needs to be distinguished from other causes of AV dissociation such as complete heart block.

Sinus rhythm usually returns by the second or third postoperative week, but late abnormalities of sinus node function of both the recipient and the donor atrium occur. This has been demonstrated in a

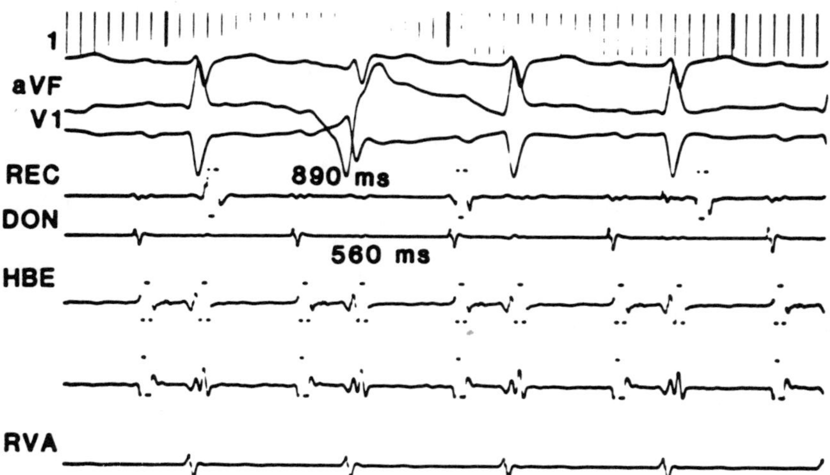

Figure 4: *Representative tracing from electrophysiologic study. The donor cycle length is 560 msec (rate 107 beats/min). Each atrial electrogram is followed by a QRS complex, best seen in either the surface leads or in the RVA. The recipient cycle length is longer, 890 msec, and has no relationship to QRS complexes. REC = recipient; DON = donor; HBE = His bundle electrogram; RVA = right ventricular apex.*

large adult series by Bexton et al., who found 4/14 donor and 6/10 recipient sinus nodes electrophysiologically abnormal.[20] In 6 of our patients who had full electrophysiologic studies, 3/6 had an abnormal donor sinus node. Two of these had prolonged sinus node recovery times greater than 525 msec and one was in junctional rhythm (Table 5). Two patients had implantation of permanent pacemakers. One had persistent slow junctional rhythm in the early postoperative period and required a pacemaker for augmentation of cardiac output. He has subsequently remained in a stable junctional rhythm. One other patient had prolonged sinus pauses greater than 3 sec by ambulatory monitoring and a markedly prolonged sinus node recovery time (Table 5). She received a pacemaker prophylactically 18 months following transplantation.

Although recipient sinus nodes can be abnormal, they remain electrically separate from the donor heart. These abnormalities, therefore, do not carry clinical significance. Because the neural connections are intact, however, they do provide the basis for determining the contribution of the nervous system to electrophysiologic function. Recipient sinus nodes were abnormal in 2/6 of our patients. One was in atrial flutter, unresponsive to overdrive pacing. Another recipient atrium had no evidence of electrical activity. There have been rare reports of synchronization of donor and recipient atrial activity but the mechanism of this is unclear.[21]

The autonomic nervous system appears to have little influence on the electrophysiologic function of the remainder of the atrioventricular conduction system. Six of our patients had full evaluation of atrial, AV

Table 5. Donor and Recipient Sinus Node Function in Six Transplant Patients

	Donor		Recipient	
Patient	CSNRT (msec)	SACT (msec)	CSNRT (msec)	SACT (msec)
SR	300	220	240	170
LC	2,180*	1,000*	130	110
JS	280	160	No electrogram*	
SD	580*	220	Flutter*	
TP	Junctional*		300	220
TT	404	140	115	100

CSNRT = corrected sinus node recovery time; SACT = sinoatrial conduction time; * = abnormal result.

nodal, and ventricular electrophysiologic function. Atrial and ventricular refractory periods were normal. AV nodal function was only mildly abnormal in one patient. With the introduction of single and double premature stimulation, no atrial or ventricular arrhythmias were inducible. These findings are similar to the findings in the innervated heart. Therefore, the resting electrophysiologic function of the atrioventricular conduction system in the transplanted heart is independent of the autonomic nervous system. Similar findings have been reported in adult patients.[22]

Response to Drugs

The response of the recipient and donor heart to various chronotropic and inotropic drugs varies. These drugs generally exert their effects either by modifying the parasympathetic and sympathetic nervous systems or by direct interaction with receptors on cardiac cells. Drugs that block the parasympathetic or sympathetic nervous systems will have no effect on the donor, but will affect the recipient normally. An example of this is seen with administration of atropine. Atropine has anticholinergic properties and exerts its major effect on the sinus and AV nodes by blocking the inhibitory response of the vagus. Sinus node function is enhanced, resulting in tachycardia, and AV nodal conduction improves. In the recipient sinus node there is an increase in rate, but there is no effect on the donor sinus node. Because the donor sinus node is unaffected, there is no increase in the ventricular response. Thus, atropine has no clinical effect on the transplanted heart. On the other hand, isoproterenol acts by interacting directly with beta receptors on the heart. It is a pure beta agonist and causes an increase in heart rate. Because of its direct action, it affects the recipient and donor heart similarly and can therefore be used in the posttransplant period. Any other drug, such as digoxin, that acts primarily by blocking the nervous system will have little use in the transplanted patient.

Arrhythmias and Sudden Death

One may speculate on the relationship of sinus node dysfunction to arrhythmia and sudden death. In adults, both supraventricular and ventricular arrhythmias occur in the early and late posttransplant period.[23,24] The first appearance of an arrhythmia may be the first sign of acute rejection. We were only able to correlate arrhythmia with rejection in one patient. This consisted of PAC, PVC, and atrial flutter in a 5-month-old infant. Complex ventricular arrhythmias may appear with accelerated atherosclerosis and sudden death, although this has not been seen in the pediatric population. Although we have had no instances of sudden death, one death was complicated by arrhythmias. This patient was an 11-year-old girl who demonstrated early sinus node dysfunction with junctional rhythm but returned to sinus rhythm by 2 weeks. Ambulatory monitoring revealed PAC without sinus bradycardia. Eight months following transplantation, a cyclosporine-related seizure occurred requiring cardiopulmonary resuscitation. Atrial flutter and ventricular tachycardia were problematic terminal events. Her autopsy showed no evidence of treatable rejection and coronary atherosclerosis was not severe. Longer follow-up with periodic ambulatory monitoring is necessary for further correlation.

The mechanism of sudden death, a known occurrence in many series, remains unclear, but arrhythmias are always suspect in these cases. Sudden death following transplantation may be multifactorial. Because transplanted hearts are denervated, they may have unstable escape pacemakers. Patients with sinus node dysfunction are therefore at risk and should be followed closely for signs of an unstable rhythm. Although we have seen no cases of accelerated atherosclerosis, this is a reported occurrence in children. Angina pectoris does not occur because of the denervated state. Frequent coronary arteriograms may be the only way of identifying those patients at risk. Longer follow-up with periodic ambulatory monitoring may optimize management of this unique patient population.

References

1. Schroeder JS: Hemodynamic performance of the human transplanted heart. Transplant Proc 1979, 9:304.
2. Greenberg ML, Uretsky BF, Reddy PS, et al: Long-term hemodynamic follow-up of cardiac transplant patients treated with cyclosporine and prednisone. Circulation 1985, 71:487.
3. Dietz RR, Patton DD, Copeland JG, et al: Characteristics of the transplanted heart in the radionuclide ventriculogram. J Heart Transplant 1986, 5:113.
4. Pflugfelder PW, Purves PD, McKenzie FN, et al: Cardiac dynamics during supine exercise in cyclosporine-treated orthotopic heart transplant

recipients: Assessment by radionuclide angiography. J Am Coll Cardiol 1987, 10:336.

5. Borow KM, Neumann A, Arensman FW, et al: Left ventricular contractility and contractile reserve in humans after cardiac transplantation. Circulation 1985, 71:866.
6. Young JB, Leon CA, Short HD III, et al: Evolution of hemodynamics after orthotopic heart and heart-lung transplantation: Early restrictive patterns persisting in occult fashion. J Heart Transplant 1987, 6:34.
7. Frist WH, Stinson EB, Oyer PE, et al: Long-term hemodynamic results after cardiac transplantation. J Thorac Cardiovasc Surg 1987, 94:685.
8. Bhatia SJS, Kirshenbaum JM, Shemin RJ, et al: Time course of resolution of pulmonary hypertension and right ventricular remodeling after orthotopic cardiac transplantation. Circulation 1987, 76:819.
9. Lewen MK, Bryg RJ, Miller LW, et al: Tricuspid regurgitation by Doppler echocardiography after orthotopic cardiac transplantation. Am J Cardiol 1987, 59:1371.
10. Pahl E, Fricker FJ, Trento A, et al. Late follow-up of children after heart transplantation. Transplant Proc 1988, 2O(Suppl I):743.
11. Stevenson LW, Dadourian BJ, Kobashigawa J, et al: Mitral regurgitation after cardiac transplantation. Am J Cardiol 1987, 60:119.
12. Stinson EB, Griepp RB, Schroeder JS, et al: Hemodynamic observations one and two years after cardiac transplantation in man. Circulation 1972, 45:1183.
13. Pope S, Stinson E, Daughters G, et al: Exercise response of the denervated heart in long-term cardiac transplant recipients. Am J Cardiol 1980, 46:213.
14. Savin W, Hashell W, Schroeder J, et al: Cardiorespiratory responses of cardiac transplant patients to graded, symptom-limited exercise. Circulation 1980, 62:55.
15. Ingels N, Ricci D, Daughters G, et al: Effects of heart rate augmentation on left ventricular volumes and cardiac output of the transplanted human heart. Circulation 1977, 56(Suppl II):32.
16. Jose AD: Effect of combined sympathetic and parasympathetic blockade on heart rate and cardiac function in man. Am J Cardiol 1966, 18:476.
17. Desai JW, Scheinman MM, Strauss HC, et al: Electrophysiologic effects of combined autonomic blockade in patients with sinus node disease. Circulation 1981, 63:953.
18. Alboni P, Malcarne C, Pedroni P, et al: Electrophysiology of normal sinus node with and without autonomic blockade. Circulation 1982, 65:1236.
19. Mackintosh AF, Carmichael DJ, Wren C, et al: Sinus node function in first three weeks after cardiac transplantation. Br Heart J 1982, 48:584.
20. Bexton R, Nathan AW, Hellestrand K, et al: Sinoatrial function after cardiac transplantation. J Am Coll Cardiol 1984, 3:712.
21. Bexton RS, Hellestrand KJ, Cory-Peace R, et al: Unusual atrial potentials in a transplant recipient: Possible synchronization between donor and recipient atria. J Electrocardiol 1983, 16:313.

22. Bexton R, Nathan A, Hellestrand J, et al: The electrophysiologic characteristics of the transplanted human heart. Am Heart J 1984, 107:1.
23. Schroeder J, Berke D, Graham A, et al: Arrhythmias after cardiac transplantation. Am J Cardiol 1974, 33:604.
24. Romhilt D, Doyle M, Sagar K, et al: Prevalence and significance of arrhythmias in long-term survivors of cardiac transplantation. Circulation 1982, 66(Suppl I):219.

Chapter 15

Assessing the Results of Heart Transplantation in Children: Morbidity, Mortality, and Quality of Life

David Baum, Daniel Bernstein, and Vaughn Starnes

Background

Heart transplantation is a lifesaving therapeutic modality for carefully selected young people. We routinely consider it for patients with end-stage cardiac disorders for whom there is no medical or surgical alternative. Although these patients are usually greatly improved postoperatively, their subsequent health and way of life are greatly influenced by the threat of allograft rejection and management of the rejection process. The purpose of this discussion is to provide a description of the benefits and liabilities of heart transplantation in children. Much of this information was garnered from the experience at the Stanford University Medical Center.

Forty-nine young people received heart transplants at Stanford over a 14-year period beginning in late 1974. At the time of transplant, their ages ranged between 5 months and 18 years. One-third of the patients were less than 9 years of age at the time of transplant, the great majority of these less than 5 years. Immunosuppression prior to December 1980 consisted of azathioprine and corticosteroids. This small group has remained on the same regimen. Patients transplanted after 1980 received cyclosporine in addition to azathioprine and corti-

From *Heart Transplantation in Children,* edited by Jeffrey M. Dunn, M.D. and Richard M. Donner, M.D.

costeroids. Follow-up of all patients has given us more than 150 patient-years of posttransplant experience.

Outcome

Realizing that life expectancy for young patients accepted for transplant is unlikely to be more than 6–12 months, much has been gained from the procedure in terms of survival. Analysis of Stanford's pediatric data revealed a cumulative survival of 77% for 1 year, 73% for 3 years, and 65% for 5 years. More than one-fourth of our patients have lived for more than 5 years. Two of our earliest patients are alive and doing well 11 years after their initial procedure.

Management advances made during the past 14 years have improved diagnostic techniques, immunosuppressive therapy, and the handling of side effects. Diagnosis and treatment have become more aggressive. As a result of this progress, survival has been prolonged, quality of life has been made better, hospitalization has become shorter and less frequent, and costs have been contained.

Benefits derived from heart transplantation were apparent within a short period after operation. Extubation, and subsequent oral feeding, and ambulation usually followed within a week. For those who did not encounter significant complications, marked improvement continued, and patients gained added strength and exercise capacity. At discharge, comparison of pre- and posttransplant conditions invariably revealed pronounced symptomatic improvement, even in those patients whose postoperative courses were difficult. With encouragement, patients and their families were able to obtain near normal lives. Patients returned to school and participated in physical education; they developed renewed interest in social and extracurricular activities. Only a few restrictions were advised. Patients were asked to avoid close contact with infected individuals. Low cholesterol diets, limiting excessive caloric intake, and excluding added salt were recommended. Sexually active girls were urged to use contraceptives because of the potential adverse effects of immunosuppression and necessary diagnostic x-ray on the fetus. No limitations were placed on physical activities.

Despite its great benefits, heart transplantation has not been without drawbacks related to potential complications of rejection and its management. Although these drawbacks do not overshadow the advantages of the procedure, they are of sufficient importance to require elaboration.

Rejection

Rejection is the result of a complex interaction between the recipient's immunologic system and the cardiac allograft. Of the rejection responses, acute rejection is by far the most common. Clinically, it may appear as soon as the end of the first postoperative week. Rejection, in this case, is mediated by both cellular and humoral immune responses.

Despite improved immunosuppressive regimens, acute rejection remained a lifelong threat. For our pediatric transplantation patients, the risk of rejection was highest in the first 3 months after transplantation. Three-fourths of the patients experienced at least one episode of rejection during this period, with the majority during the first month. After the early months, patients remained at risk for rejection, albeit to a lesser extent.

Clinically, acute rejection was suspected with the appearance of any of the following: arrhythmia, unexplained tachycardia, gallop rhythm, reduced ECG voltage, increasing pericardial effusion, and increasing heart size. Echocardiographically demonstrable reduction of diastolic function also prompted suspicion of the rejection process; however, impaired systolic function became apparent only when acute rejection was more advanced. The use of cyclosporine modified the rejection process, causing it to be indolent and clinically subtle. Thus, most rejection episodes in recent years were not associated with clinical findings. Because clinical detection of acute rejection has not been sufficiently sensitive in the view of Stanford physicians, endomyocardial biopsy was performed for monitoring the rejection process and confirmation of its diagnosis.

Acute rejection was managed with medical therapy in most instances. In the early transplant months, it was treated with a 3-day course of intravenous methylprednisolone. Later, acute rejection was treated with an increase in prednisone dosage, which was subsequently tapered over a matter of weeks. Whenever acute rejection was diagnosed and treated, subsequent management was monitored primarily by endomyocardial biopsy. When steroid therapy was unsuccessful, antithymocyte globulin, the monoclonal antibody OKT3, and total body irradiation were used to suppress rejection. In 8% of our young patients, acute rejection was unresponsive to medical management and retransplantation was required. In such cases, it was invariably necessary within the first 6 months after the initial transplant procedure. Following retransplantation, the rejection rate increased for a few months and then returned to a lower level.

Acute rejection was an uncommon source of morbidity and mortality in the pediatric age group. It has become less of a problem since cyclosporine was added to the immunosuppressive regimen. Both morbidity and mortality were far more often the result of complications secondary to the management of acute rejection rather than from the rejection process itself.

Infection

Infection was a serious complication of chronic immunosuppression in children. It was the most common reason for prolonged hospitalization and, by far, the most common cause of death in Stanford's young heart transplant patients. Two-thirds of the total pediatric mortality was due to infection. The great majority of these infection-related deaths occurred within 6 months of receiving a cardiac allograft.

The incidence of infection was highest in the first postoperative month when the marked risk of rejection required the greatest degree of immunosuppression. After the first month, the rate of infection fell and by the end of the third postoperative month, it plateaued. By that time, two-thirds of the patients had experienced at least one significant infection. Although the rate of infection was low after the early postoperative months, infection remained a lifelong threat. In patients who were retransplanted, however, the risk increased again and was directly time-related to the most recent allograft.

Although minor upper respiratory tract infections occurred and resolved without particular difficulty, it was disease caused by opportunistic infections that produced morbidity and mortality in young patients given heart transplants. Bacterial infections were common in Stanford's pediatric heart transplant population, causing 45% of major infections. Enterococci, klebsiella, pseudomonas, serratia, and staphylococcus were most frequently isolated. The lung was the most common site of infection; the urinary tract and blood stream were also frequently involved.

Viral infections also were common, causing 40% of significant infective episodes. The majority, however, were not serious. Mucocutaneous herpes simplex was the predominant viral infection. Two other members of the herpesvirus group, cytomegalovirus and varicella-zoster virus, caused more serious infections. The cytomegalovirus was a particular problem for two reasons. After a period of latency, institution of immunosuppression resulted in reactivation of the organism and serious infection. More often, cytomegaloviral infection developed in seronegative recipients receiving cardiac allografts from infected donors. Under these circumstances, infection was particularly virulent because of immunosuppression. Serious pulmonary involvement was common, and the infection often became disseminated and led to death.

Fungal infections were less common, causing about 10% of significant infections. These infections often were disseminated and particularly difficult to control. Although etiologic agents in a relatively small proportion of infections, fungi played a primary role in over half the mortality secondary to infection in Stanford's pediatric heart transplant group.

Two other organisms were sources of opportunistic infection. *Pneumocystis carinii* was an uncommon cause of pneumonia in our patients. In two cases, it produced considerable morbidity, but no mortality. There was one nocardial infection of the lung from which the patient recovered.

Coronary Artery Disease

Coronary artery disease has been a major cause of graft failure in long-term survivors of heart transplantation. In adults, it has been observed in 36% of recipients who survived at least 1 year following the procedure.[1] The disorder was found in 23% of our young patients surviving a similar length of time. Allograft coronary artery disease appeared unrelated to the recipient's age, sex, or preoperative cardiac diagnosis. We have seen this coronary vascular abnormality in children less than 5 years of age. Furthermore, observations in adults suggest that graft coronary artery disease does not seem related to the number of rejection episodes, the amount of corticosteroids given, or donor–recipient matching.[1] Recipient serum lipid profiles have been unrevealing except for a minor increase in triglyceride levels in patients developing graft coronary artery disease.[1]

The coronary disorder found in cardiac allografts is unusual in several respects.[2] Rarely, it can begin within a few weeks of transplantation and proceed with sufficient rapidity to cause coronary occlusion in just a few months. More often, the course is prolonged. Extensive coronary artery involvement requiring retransplantation, however, can occur within a few years of receiving a heart transplant.

There are two types of anatomic abnormality.[2,3] One category is quite similar to naturally occurring atherosclerosis. It produces discrete and tubular stenoses largely in the proximal and mid portions of the major epicardial coronary vessels. Focal intimal plaques, destruction of the internal elastic lamina, and calcification are common. Thus, it may be indistinguishable from the atherosclerotic coronary artery disease usually associated with aging. The second type of abnormality involves the secondary and tertiary vessels, including intramuscular branches of the major epicardial arteries. It is associated with diffuse concentric narrowing and gradual tapering of distal branches. Angiographically, these narrowed vessels are irregular or poorly visualized; interval occlusion and distal obliteration are common. When allograft coronary artery disease occurs, it typically includes both categories of abnormality.

Clinical recognition of coronary artery disease in the young transplant recipient is difficult because the graft is denervated. As a result, the patient does not experience typical anginal pain and cannot communicate symptoms of myocardial ischemia. ECG, nuclear angiography, and treadmill testing are insufficiently sensitive to be relied upon for detection of the disorder. If graft coronary artery disease proceeds unrecognized, progressive myocardial ischemia may develop, producing infarction, ventricular arrhythmia, congestive heart failure, and even sudden death. Therefore, annual coronary angiography is performed for detection and monitoring of this potential complication. Even though we have not recognized coronary disease angiographically in children within the first 2 years of transplantation, we recommend beginning annual studies within the first year in order to provide the necessary baseline for future comparisons.

Available medical therapies have proven unsatisfactory in the management of allograft coronary artery disease.[4] The character of the disorder does not make it amenable to coronary angioplasty or coronary bypass procedures. Preventative measures, such as dietary restrictions and antiplatelet agents, have so far not proven efficacious.

Repeat heart transplantation has been the only effective treatment for severe graft coronary artery disease.[4] It is performed electively when extensive coronary artery involvement is demonstrated angiographically. Thus far, three individuals who received allografts as children were advised to undergo retransplantation because of coronary artery disease. Two were successfully retransplanted: the first, 11 years and the second, 2 years following their initial transplant procedures. The third, advised to undergo retransplantation 3½ years after receiving an allograft, refused. He died of acute myocardial infarction 4 months later.

Malignancy

Cancer is far more common in patients who are immunosuppressed, occurring 100 times more often than in the population as a whole.[5] Non-Hodgkins lymphoma is particularly prevalent among immunosuppressed individuals and has been described in 7% of adult heart transplant patients.[4] Therefore, it was not unexpected that 10% of our young patients developed malignancies and all but one was found to have a lymphoma. The exception was a child with hepatic carcinoma.

Half of this pediatric group with malignancies became symptomatic, whereas in the other half, malignancy was an unexpected finding at autopsy. It was the cause of death in only one case, a patient symptomatic with lymphoma. This individual developed his primary lesion at the muscular site where antithymocyte globulin was previously administered. Death occurred despite chemotherapy. A second patient, an infant, was found to have widespread symptomatic lymphoproliferative disease less than 6 months after receiving a cardiac allograft. Because Epstein-Barr viral genome was detected in biopsy material from the tumor, he was treated with a reduction in immunosuppressive therapy and with acyclovir. Subsequently, the disorder regressed and he is now free of disease 18 months later. The third symptomatic patient had a central nervous system lymphoma treated with radiation and has been free of disease for more than 10 years.

Drug Side Effects

Corticosteroids

Corticosteroids are associated with a number of undesirable side effects. That of growth impairment is especially relevant in the care of children. A reduction in growth was found in many of our pediatric patients and was more apparent in individuals receiving steroids at ages when growth was expected to accelerate. The cushingoid state was prevalent, although varying in degree, and increased appetite and excessive weight gain were also common problems. These side effects were particularly troublesome in teenagers because of their great concern with physical appearance. As a result, counseling was occasionally required. In patients receiving steroids without cyclosporine, only occasional blood pressure elevations were observed, and these blood pressure disturbances often responded satisfactorily to the administration of diuretics. X-ray evidence of bone demineralization was another complication. In two patients, aseptic necrosis of weight-bearing joints was observed, but pathologic fractures did not occur. Because of the risk for peptic ulcer, antacids were given prophylactically on a routine basis. Personality lability and headache were infrequent and could not be specifically ascribed to the steroids. Whereas relatively mild carbohydrate intolerance was found there was no need for insulin administration. Because of their many unwanted effects, considerable effort was made to minimize the amount of steroids administered.

Azathioprine

Although azathioprine was routinely given in dosages aimed at maintaining the white blood cell count between 4,000–5,000/10^3mm, leukopenia and, less often, thrombocytopenia were observed. In the presence of viral infections, especially those due to cytomegalovirus, bone marrow suppression was more frequent. Generally, this response to azathioprine was dose-dependent and reversible. Hepatotoxicity, manifested by alterations in liver function tests, was occasionally observed but was minor. Liver function abnormalities also were reversed by lowering drug dosage. Nausea, vomiting, and abdominal discomfort have been described, but did not occur in our patients.

Cyclosporine

Cyclosporine is responsible for a number of side effects.[6] Because of some of cyclosporine's complications, the dosage has been reduced from that used after its initial introduction in 1980. The renal and neurologic complications can be of great consequence. Although kidney dysfunction was frequent in our patients, it usually was not severe. It was made evident by elevation of serum creatinine and blood urea nitrogen levels and reduction in creatinine clearance. In the pediatric patients, these laboratory changes usually developed within a year of beginning cyclosporine administration. In most, these laboratory values stabilized after a year or so. Although dosage adjustment was required, it was rarely necessary to discontinue cyclosporine administration because of complications due to the drug. Rarely, prolonged administration of cyclosporine can produce progressive kidney damage as it did in one young patient after 7 years. He has required renal dialysis during the past year and is now awaiting renal transplantation. Headache and fine tremor have been sources of complaint, but no more serious abnormalities have been reported. None of the young persons in the Stanford Transplant Program experienced a seizure.

Hypertension of varying severity was a particularly frequent management problem in young persons receiving cyclosporine. Invariably, blood pressure elevation began within 1 or 2 weeks of introducing the drug and, unless treated, continued. Both systolic and diastolic pressures were elevated. Generally, hypertension became more severe when large amounts of steroids were used for treatment of acute rejection. Diuretic therapy was rarely sufficient for blood pressure control. More often, two, and sometimes three, medications were required to lower blood pressure to acceptable levels. One patient developed a hypertensive crisis and coma that responded to intravenous antihypertensive therapy.

Other side effects were annoying, although of lesser consequence. Hirsutism was frequent, requiring use of a depilatory agent in some adolescent girls. Gingival hyperplasia also was common, and in some, periodontal surgery was necessary. There have been occasional minor abnormalities of liver function, which regressed with reduction of cyclosporine dosage. Nausea and vomiting, cramps, gynecomastia, anemia and thrombocytopenia are said to occur, but were not found in our patients.

Perspective

The overall experience among Stanford's young heart transplantation patients has been extremely positive. Long-term survival represents a reasonable expectation. Despite certain limitations, the quality of life for surviving patients is good. Our long-term results appear to satisfy both patients and their families. In addition, our results continue to improve. Therefore, we believe that the net result is sufficiently beneficial to recommend heart transplantation for selected pediatric patients with end-stage heart disease and no medical or surgical alternative.

References

1. Gao SZ, Schroeder JS, Alderman EL, et al: Clinical and laboratory correlates of accelerated coronary artery disease in the cardiac transplant patient. Circulation 1987, 76(Suppl V):56.
2. Billingham ME: Cardiac transplant atherosclerosis. Transplant Proc 1987, 19(Suppl 5):19.
3. Gao SZ, Alderman EL, Schroeder JS, et al: Accelerated coronary vascular disease in the heart transplant patient: Coronary arteriographic findings. J Am Coll Cardiol 1988, 12:334.
4. Hunt SA: Complications of heart transplantation. Heart Transplant 1983, 3:70.
5. Penn I: Depressed immunity and the development of cancer. Clin Exp Immunol 1981, 46:459.
6. Kahan BD: Immunosuppressive therapy with cyclosporine for cardiac transplantation. Circulation 1987, 75:40.

Chapter 16

Experience with Heart Transplantation in Children at the University of Pittsburgh and Children's Hospital

F. Jay Fricker, Alfredo Trento, Bartley Griffith, Robert L. Hardesty, Lee B. Beerman, Kathy Lawrence, Elfriede Pahl, Henry T. Bahnson, J. R. Zuberbuhler

Introduction

The first pediatric heart transplantation at Children's Hospital of Pittsburgh was performed in February 1982. To date, 30 patients, age range 5 months to 17 years, have undergone heart, heart–liver, or heart–lung transplantation. Seventeen patients are currently alive, and 10 of those patients have survived longer than 1 year after transplantation.

Patient Population and Recipient Selection

Dilated cardiomyopathy and palliated congenital heart disease with irreversible myocardial dysfunction are the major indications for heart transplantation in children.[1] There were 22 patients receiving orthotopic heart transplants. Thirteen of those patients had a diagnosis

From *Heart Transplantation in Children*, edited by Jeffrey M. Dunn, M.D. and Richard M. Donner, M.D.

of idiopathic cardiomyopathy, seven had congenital heart disease, and two had severe viral myocarditis. One patient with a restrictive cardiomyopathy and elevated pulmonary vascular resistance underwent heterotopic heart transplantation. Three children underwent combined heart–liver transplantation, two for primary hypercholesterolemia with ischemic cardiomyopathy and one with intrahepatic biliary atresia and a dilated cardiomyopathy.

We have a limited experience with heart–lung transplantation in children. Four procedures have been done: two for primary pulmonary hypertension, another for pulmonary vascular disease secondary to congenital heart disease, and one for primary desquamative interstitial pneumonitis.

Selection of recipients for cardiac transplantation has an obvious impact on survival. Up until this time, we have not turned down any possible heart transplant recipient if we thought there was any chance of success. Patients with significant end-organ dysfunction, pulmonary embolus and infarction, elevated pulmonary vascular resistance, and pulmonary artery anatomy that required reconstruction at the time of the transplant have all been done with an adverse impact on early morbidity and mortality. In view of the current shortage of donor organs, this approach may not be appropriate in any transplantation program.

Outcome

Figure 1 depicts the survival curve for 30 patients receiving heart, heart–liver, and heart–lung transplantation over the past 5 years. There was a high early mortality (30%). Major causes of death in this group were primary organ failure (3), technical problems related to pulmonary artery anatomy and complex congenital heart disease (2), and infection (2). Elevated pulmonary vascular resistance, intracranial hemorrhage, and poor donor selection for a heart–lung transplant recipient each accounted for one early death. Three late deaths were all due to acute and chronic rejection. Two of these patients had extensive coronary atherosclerosis, as well as chronic myocardial inflammation and fibrosis. Currently there are 10 children who have survived beyond 1 year following transplantation, including 1 patient who received a heart–liver transplantation and 1 with a heart–lung transplant. The longest survivor is now 5 years from transplantation with

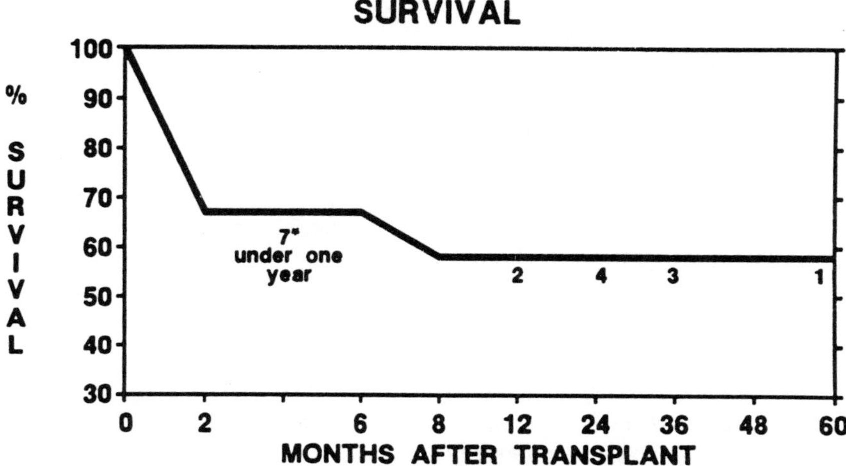

Figure 1: *Survival of 30 children receiving heart, heart–liver, and heart–lung transplant.*

three others surviving three years, four surviving two years and two patients alive one year after operation. Seven recipients are less than 1 year after transplantation surgery.

Immunosuppression and Rejection

Immune suppression therapy in children and changes in those regimens have evolved along with our adult experience.[2,3] Although cyclosporine and prednisone were initially used successfully, rejection became the prime cause of death and, therefore, antithymocyte globulin (ATG) was added as rescue therapy for acute rejection. Chronic immunosuppressive regimens subsequently added azathioprine to cyclosporine and prednisone to minimize the nephrotoxicity of cyclosporine. In late 1986, we began to use ATG prophylactically for the first 3 to 5 days following transplantation. Current immunosuppression utilizes azathioprine (4 mg/kg) preoperatively, Solu-Medrol (20 mg/kg) intraoperatively, and prophylactic antithymocyte globulin (ATG) (1.5 mg/kg/day) for 3–5 days postoperatively. Cyclosporine, prednisone and azathioprine are used for chronic immune suppression. Cyclosporine dose has varied between 4 and 20 mg/kg/day while initially maintaining whole blood radioimmunoassay RIA cyclosporine level above 700 ng/mL. After 6 months, cyclosporine dose is decreased to target levels of 500 ng/mL by RIA and 150–250 ng/mL by the high-performance liquid chromatography (HPLC) method. Prednisone dose has varied between 0.1 and 0.3 mg/kg/day.

Rejection episodes are nearly a universal phenomenon in the first 3 months following heart transplantation in children. Analysis of rejection events demonstrates that only three children (18%) have been completely free of treated rejection episodes since their heart transplant. All three children received prophylactic ATG as initial immunosuppression. The frequency of rejection episodes has also been substantially reduced in this group of patients. There were two episodes of serious and symptomatic rejection that occurred 15 months and 2 years following transplantation. Both were associated with reduction or discontinuation of corticosteroids. This has emphasized the importance of periodic endomyocardial biopsies late after transplantation, particularly when changes in immunosuppression are undertaken.

Rejection in heart–lung transplant recipients was more difficult to diagnose with assurance. Rejection was asynchronous, primarily with lung rather than heart involved. A change on chest X-ray or decrease in systemic oxygen saturation generally warranted treatment.

Complications of Immunosuppression

Infection

Infection remains a significant early complication in cyclosporine-treated transplantation recipients.[4] Early bacterial infection with *Pseudomonas aeruginosa* accounted for two deaths. One patient with mediastinitis and another with pneumonia and endocarditis had both been reoperated on because of bleeding following transplantation. Another patient recovered from a *Serratia marcescens* pneumonia, peritonitis, and mediastinitis.

Serious viral infections have generally occurred greater than 1 month following transplantation. One heart–lung recipient died after cytomegalovirus pneumonia, and a second heart–lung transplant recipient had a complicated course following primary Epstein-Barr virus infection in her lung.

Prophylactic treatment for *Pneumocystis carinii* infection has not routinely been given to our heart transplant recipients and we have seen only one case of pneumocystis pneumonia. This infection occurred in a child after repeated increases in his immunosuppressive regimen to control rejection. He did survive this infection, but subsequently died of graft rejection.

Late bacterial and viral infections have been relatively infrequent. Sinusitis, otitis, urinary tract infection with common organisms, and herpetic gingivostomatitis have all been seen without any serious sequelae.

Hypertension

Systemic hypertension is by far the major hemodynamic abnormality following transplantation and is clearly related, in part, to cyclosporine therapy.[5] Essentially all recipients have required antihypertensive therapy and 7 of 10 patients that have survived longer than 1 year are currently on chronic antihypertensive regimens. The mechanism of hypertension is unclear, but is thought to be related to renal vasoconstriction caused by cyclosporine. Clinically, the hypertension is characterized by a lack of diurnal decrease in blood pressure. Hypertension has been difficult to treat, and therapeutic regimens usually begin with diuretics and angiotensin blocking agents. Recently, long-acting calcium channel blocking agents, such as verapamil and sustained-release combination β- and α-adrenergic blocking agents have also been helpful.

Renal function

Careful monitoring of renal function is necessary because of the known nephrotoxic effects of cyclosporine.[6] We monitor whole blood cyclosporine levels by both radioimmunoassay (RIA) and high-performance liquid chromatography (HPLC) methods at frequent intervals. Cyclosporine dosages are variable and adjusted to maintain HPLC cyclosporine levels between 150 and 250 ng/mL depending on time elapsed since transplantation. We have used serum creatinine as an estimate of the glomerular filtration rate (GFR) in these children because of the difficulty in obtaining complete and accurately timed urine collections for creatinine clearance (Fig. 2).[7] Serum creatinines generally return to normal in the first month following transplantation,

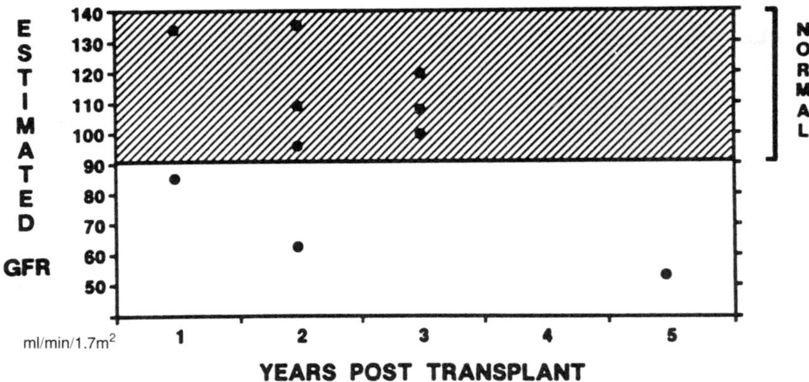

Figure 2: *Estimated GFR in 10 patients surviving longer than 1 year since transplant surgery. (From Schwartz GJ, Haycock GB, Ejelman CM, et al. Pediatrics 1976, 58:259.*[7]*)*

due to the improvement of myocardial function. Reviewing renal function in those patients surviving longer than 1 year after transplantation, we see uniform and substantial rise in serum creatinine in most patients. Over the subsequent years, serum creatinine has tended to remain stable except in our longest surviving transplant recipient. In this adolescent, serum creatinine reached a peak of just over 2 mg% and necessitated a substantial reduction in cyclosporine dose and the addition of azathioprine to her immunosupression regimens. There is also recent evidence that serum creatinine and creatinine clearance do not accurately reflect cyclosporine nephrotoxicity.[8] The abnormalities in serum creatinine that we have seen are significant, and we are concerned that long-term use of cyclosporine may cause progressive renal dysfunction in children.

Growth

We have assessed growth and weight gain in children surviving longer than 1 year since year transplant and have shown that linear growth has been maintained in 8 of 10 of these patients. In contrast, the majority of patients have shown a marked increase in weight, with only four patients remaining on the same weight percentile (Fig. 3). At

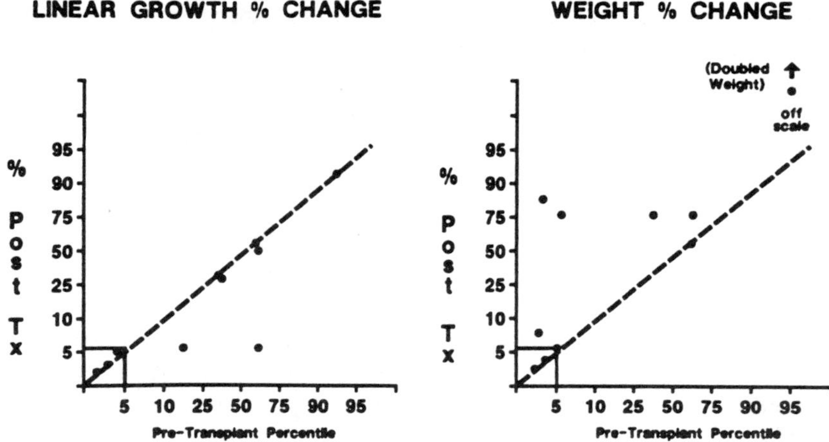

Figure 3: *Pre-and posttransplant linear growth and weight percentiles in 10 pediatric patients surviving longer than 1 year after transplantation surgery.*

their latest follow-up visit, six patients have crossed weight percentiles and one patient is morbidly obese.

Current status

In general, most transplant recipients have returned to age-appropriate activities with some notable exceptions. The patient receiving a heterotopic heart transplant for restrictive cardiomyopathy remains symptomatic because pulmonary vascular resistance has not dropped as expected and limits his cardiac output and exercise tolerance. The child with desquamative interstitial pneumonia who received a heart/lung transplant nearly 2 years ago had an excellent initial year. She subsequently has developed chronic airway rejection and is currently symptomatic with components of both restrictive and obstructive lung disease, as well as recurrent Pseudomonas bronchitis.

Graft function has been assessed by echocardiography and radionuclide angiography. Echocardiographic dimensions and systolic function are normal, except for mild increases in myocardial wall thickness. Radionuclide ejection fraction (LVEF) is in the normal range (LVEF >50% in all patients 1 to 5 years after heart transplant).

Heart rhythm has been monitored with 24-hour-Holter monitoring. Two children have evidence of AV node disease. One adolescent had a severe rejection episode 15 months after transplantation, resulting in intermittent complete heart block that required permanent pacemaker insertion.

Coronary arteriography is part of our long-term, follow-up monitoring, and all coronary angiograms have been normal with the exception of one adolescent who has minor lesions in his left anterior descending coronary artery. This same patient has systemic hypertension, hypercholesterolemia, and is morbidly obese.

We continue to be concerned about late effects of cyclosporine on blood pressure and kidney function. Hypertension has been a long-term problem with the majority of patients requiring antihypertensive therapy. At least four patients have significantly abnormal renal function as estimated from serum creatinine. If serum creatinine is shown to underestimate the degree of nephrotoxicity from cyclosporine, significant reduction in cyclosporine dose will be necessary to prevent chronic renal disease in these patients. Once a patient has doubled serum creatinine, efforts should be made to substantially reduce cyclosporine dose and add azathioprine to that patient's regimen.

In summary, we believe that heart transplantation is an acceptable option for children with terminal heart and heart–lung disease who have no other therapeutic option. Future advances in immunosuppression and the development of a noninvasive and accurate method of assessing rejection will allow for increased survival as well as an improved quality of life.

References

1. Pennington D, Sarafian J, Swartz M: Heart transplantation in children. J Heart Transplant 1985, 4:441.
2. Hardesty RL, Griffith BP, Debski RF, et al: Experience with cyclosporine in cardiac transplantation. Transplant Proc 1983, 15:(Suppl I)2553.
3. Griffith BP, Hardesty RL, Thompson ME, et al: Cardiac transplantation with cyclosporine—The Pittsburgh experience. Heart Transplant 1983, 2:251.
4. Green M, Wald E, Fricker J, et al: Infections following orthotopic heart transplant in pediatric patients. (Abstract) Presented at the 27th ICAAC. Oct. 1987, New York, N.Y.
5. Thompson ME, Shapiro AP, Johnson AM, et al: New onset of hypertension following cardiac transplantation: A preliminary report and analysis. Transplant Proc 1983, 14:(Suppl I)2573.
6. Myers BD, Ross J, Newton L, et al: Cyclosporine—Associated chronic nephropathy. N Engl J Med 1984, 311:699.

7. Schwartz GJ, Haycock GB, Ejelman CM, et al: A simple estimate of glomerular filtration rate in children derived from body length and plasma creatinine. Pediatrics 1976, 58:259.
8. Tomlanovich S, Golbetz H, Perlroth M, et al: Am J Kidney Dis 1986, 8:332.

APPENDIX A.
Preoperative Candidate Evaluation Checklist

FOR C-T OFFICE USE ONLY EVALUATION CHECKLIST FOR TRANSPLANT CANDIDATES *G26:EVALCK.R*

PATIENT NAME ______________________ REFERRING M.D. ______________________

TYPE OF TX: Heart ____ Heart/Lung ____ Single Lung ____

S.S. #: ____-__-____ D.O.B.: ___/___/___ Maiden Name: ______________

Address: ______________________ Telephone No.: (H) ( ) ____________
______________________ (W) ( ) ____________

Height: ________ Weight: ________ Age: _____ Sex: ____ Ethnic Background: __________

****

CONSULTS		Date Sent	CONSULTS		Date Sent
Cardiology -	( )	______	Oral Surgery -	( )	______
C-T Surgery -	( )	______	Social Work -	( )	______
Psychiatry -	( )	______	Dietary -	( )	______
Pulmonary *(H/L and Lung only)* -	( )	______			

****

LAB WORK	Date Sent	Result	LAB WORK	Date Sent	Result
ABO type & Screen	______	______	Virology/Serology		
3 green + 1 red (HUP 662-6010):			1. CMV	______	______
Anti-HLA Rapid Specific	______	______	2. EBV	______	______
P.R.A.	______	______	3. Toxoplasmosis	______	______
24 hr Creatinine clearance	______	______	4. HIV	______	______
Lipid Profile	______	______	5. Hepatitis B	______	______

****

SPECIAL TESTS/PROCEDURES		Date Ordered	Result
A. Heart TX Candidates:	1. Rt. Heart Catheterization	______	______
	a) $PVR = \frac{PAP - PCWP}{C.O.}$	______	______
	b) PAP	______	______
	c) PCWP	______	______
	d) $C.I. = \frac{C.O.}{BSA}$	______	______
B. Heart/Lung TX Candidates:	1. Echocardiogram	______	______
	2. PFT's, complete	______	______
	3. Sputum C&S, fungal & TB	______	______
	4. IGG, IGE	______	______
C. Cystic Fibrosis Patients Only:	1. Consult Pharmacokinetics ( )	______	______
	2. Int. PPD	______	______
	3. Ind. Calorimetry ( )	______	______
	4. HgB A_1C	______	______
	5. Room Air ABG	______	______

****

APPENDIX B.
Postoperative Patient Flow Sheet

TEMPLE UNIVERSITY HOSPITAL HEART TRANSPLANT PROGRAM

CLINICAL															CHEMISTRY						
DATE	PODAY	OUTPUT	WEIGHT Kg	TEMP	BP	HEART RATE	RHYTHM	C.O.	MAP	PAP s/d	PCWP	CVP	SVR	PVR	NA	K	CL	CO_2	BUN	CREAT	TP

Appendix B. contd.

RECIPIENT

Name____

Age__________Sex______________________________

Date of Transplant ______________________________

Blood Group __________________________________

Histocompatibility______________________________

Height ________ Weight ________________________

Titers_______CMV______ EBV______________________

CHEMISTRY											HEMATOLOGY									
ALB	INORPHOS	GLUCOSE	TBILI	INDIRBILI	ALKPHOS	AST	ALT	CPK	CPK mb	LDH	WBC	DIFFERENTIAL				HGB	HCT	PLATELETS	PT	PTT
												N	L	M	E					

Appendix B. contd.

DONOR

Age______ Sex ________________

Location ________________________

Blood Group ________________________

Pump Time ________________________

Ischemic Time ________________________

Preservation ________________________

Post/Pre Crossmatch ________________________

Titers ______ CMV ______ EBV ____________

CULTURES				THERAPY								IMMUNOLOGIC MONITORING				MYOCARDIAL BIOPSY
URINE	SPUTUM	BLOOD	OTHER	PREDNISONE	SOLUMEDROL	ATGAM	CYCLOSPORINE	OTHER DRUGS				CYCLOSPORINE				

Appendix B. contd.

COMMENTS	PLAN

APPENDIX C.
Heart Transplantation Computer Data Base


```
**************************************************
*                TEMPLE UNIVERSITY               *
*    CARDIOPULMONARY TRANSPLANTATION REGISTRY    *
**************************************************
```

PATIENT INFORMATION

Patient Name (last,first,m.): ________________
BOSS #: ________ Social Security #: __-__-____ Tx #: ____
Address: ________________
City: ________________ State: __ Zip: _____ Country: ______
Telephone-Home: __-__-____ Work: __-__-____
Date of Birth: __-__-__ Age: ___ Sex: ______ Ethnic Background: ________

Type TX: ________ PRIMARY CARDIAC DIAGNOSIS: ________________
PRIMARY PULMONARY DIAGNOSIS: ________________
Cardiomyopathy: ___ Type: ________________

Employment: ________________
Employer: ________________ Tel #: __-__-____ Contact: ________
Address: ________________ City: ________ State: __ Zip: _____
Provider-Primary: ________________ Guarantor: ________________
Address: ________________ City: ________ State: __ Zip: _____
ID #: ________ Group #: ________ Plan: ___
PreCert Contact: ________________ Tel #: __-__-____ Forms Req? ___
Deductible: ________________
Outpt Coverage: ________________
Provider-Secondary: ________________ Guarantor: ________________
Address: ________________ City: ________ State: __ Zip: _____
ID #: ________ Group #: ________ Plan: ___
PreCert Contact: ________________ Tel #: __-__-____ Forms Req? ___
Deductible: ________________
Outpt Coverage: ________________
Comments: ________________

Hospital Admitted: ________________ Transferring Hospital: ________________

Dates: Admission: __-__-__ Surgery: __-__-__ Discharge: __-__-__
LOS (PreTx): ___ LOS (PostTx): ___ LOS (Total): ___

PHYSICIANS

Referring Cardiologist: ________________
Surgeon: ________________
Asst Surgeon: ________________
Harvest Team: ________________
Surgical Asst: ________________
Perfusionist: ________________
Anesthesiologist: ________________
Referring Primary Physician: ________________

Notes: ________________

PATIENT HISTORY

Education: ____________________

Marital Status: ________

Hand Dominance _____

Date/Documented Diagnosis: __-__-__

Date/CHF 1st Episode: __-__-__

MEDICAL HISTORY

Hypertension	___	Diabetes (juvenile)	___	Diabetes (adult onset)	___
COPD	___	Renal Insufficiency	___	Alcoholism	___
CVA	___	Pulmonary Embolism	___	Deep Vein Thrombosis	___
Gout	___	Endocarditis	___	CNS Infection	___
Renal Stones	___	Acne	___	Seizure Disorder	___
Psychiatric	___	Myocardial Infarct	___	Rheumatic Heart Disease	___
Current Smoker	___	Past Smoker	___	*Smoker How Long? (yrs)	__
Oral Contracep	___	Arthritis	___	Collagen Vascular Dis	___
Ulcer Disease	___	Cancer	___	Diverticulosis	___
Drug Abuse	___	Gallbladder Disease	___	Peripheral Vas Disease	___
Cardiac Arrest	___	Respiratory Arrest	___	Other	____________

Drug Allergies: ________ ________ ________

Previous Cardiac Surgery: ___

Procedure		Date		Comps
CABG	___	__-__-__	Conduit ___	___
CABG + VR	___	__-__-__	Conduit ___	___
AVR	___	__-__-__		___
MVR	___	__-__-__		___
Multi Valves	___	__-__-__		___
Aneurysmectomy	___	__-__-__		___
Transplant	___	__-__-__		___
VSD	___	__-__-__		___
Other	____________	__-__-__		___
	____________	__-__-__		___
	____________	__-__-__		___

OTHER CARDIAC SURGERY

Congenital Surgery: ___ **Date:** ___-___-___
Procedure: ______________________________

Other Thoracic Surgery: ___ **Date:** ___-___-___
Procedure: ______________________________

Other Vascular Surgery: ___ **Date:** ___-___-___
Procedure: ______________________________

Pacemaker: ___ **Date:** ___-___-___
Type: ________________
Manufacturer: ________________
Model: ___________ **Mode:** ___-___-___
S/N: ________________

PRE-TRANSPLANT MEDICATIONS

Diuretics ___
Digitalis ___
Vasodilators ___
Beta Blockers ___
Anticoagulants ___
Inotropes-IV ___ Drug ________________
Inotropes-Oral ___
Antiarrhythmics ___
ACE Inhibitors ___
Nitrates ___
Inotrope-IV-Trial ___ Drug ________________
Other ________________
Other ________________

Obstetrical History:

Gravida __
Para __
Abortions __

Complications of Pregnancy: ___
Pre-eclampsia ___
Eclampsia ___
Other ___ Specify: ________________

RECIPIENT TRANSPLANT DATA

Type of Transplant: ____________________________

Transplant Surgery Data:

Bypass Time: ____ min X-Clamp Time: ____ min Reperfusion Time: ____ min
Patient Weight (kg): _____ BSA (M2): _____
Bypass Oxygenator: ______________________

Myocardial Protection: Cardioplegia: St Thomas: ___ Blood: ___ Cryst: ___
Volume Delivered(ml): ______
Hypothermia: Topical: ___ Systemic: ___
Temperatures: Bladder: _____ C

IABP: ___ Indication: ________________
Insertion Period: _______
Duration (hr): ____

LVAD: ___ Type: ________________
Indication: ________________
Duration: ____

RVAD: ___ Type: ________________
Indication: ________________
Duration: _____

Periop Pacing ___ Type: ________________ Mode: ______ Implant: ___

Support Medications: ___

Dobutamine	___	Dopamine	___
Epineph	___	Levophed	___
Nitropruss	___	Isuprel	___
Lidocaine	___	Pronestyl	___
NTG	___	Other __________	
Other __________		Other __________	

Anesthesia Comments: ____

Other Comments: ____
____
____

Recipient Tx Data:

Tissue Typing: **Cytotoxic Antibodies:**
B-Cells (%): _____ vs. T-Cells (%): _____

Donor/Recipient Cross Match Done: ___ Findings: ___________

ABO Blood Type: __ RH Factor: _

HLA TYPING:	Recipient	Donor
A	___/___	___/___
B	___/___	___/___
C	___/___	___/___
DR	___/___	___/___

Previous Transfusions: ___ Date: __-__-__

UNOS Data: Description of Patient at Time Of Tx:

Cat #: _ Description: _________________________

Immunosuppression:

Type: _________________________

ATGam: ___ # of Days: ___

OKT3: ___ # of Days: ___

Comment: _______________________________________

DONOR TRANSPLANT DATA

Donor's Name: ____________________________________ Age: _____ Sex: ______

Cause of Death: _________________________ Date of Death: __-__-__

Weight: ___ lb _____ kg

Blood Type: __ RH Factor: _

Ischemic Time (min): ___

Donor Locale: _________________________

Length of Time of Ventilation (days): ____

Donor Condition:

Echo Normal	___	**Mitral Valve Prolapse**	___	
Normal EKG	___	**Normal Chest X-Ray**	___	
Arrhythmia (Atrial)	___	**Inotropic Support**	___	***Hrs:___**
Steroids	___	**Mannitol**	___	
Transfusion History	___	**Other** ____________________		

Evidence of Infection:	___	**Pneumonia:**	___
		Positive Blood Culture:	___
		Positive Urine Culture:	___

Viral Titers: CMV: 1:______ EBV: 1:______ TOXO: 1:______

Viral Antibodies: CMV: ___ HAA: ___ HIV: ___ TOXO: ___

Multiorgan Harvest: ___

Organ		Harvest Team
Liver	___	_________________________
R Kidney	___	_________________________
L Kidney	___	_________________________
Pancreas	___	_________________________
Small Intestine	___	_________________________
Tissue	___	_________________________
Cornea	___	_________________________
Skin	___	_________________________
Bone/Marrow	___	_________________________
Lung	___	_________________________

PostOp Complications: ___

Surgical:	___	Reop/Bleed:	___	Organ Dysfunction:	_
		Low Cardiac Output:	___		
Infection:	___	Sternum-Deep:	___	Sternum-Super:	_
		Lines:	___	IABP/VAD/TAH:	_
Neuro:	___	Stroke-Transient:	___	Stroke-Permanent:	_
		Delirium/Confusion:	___	Neuropathy:	_
		Seizures:	___		
Arrhythmias:	___	V-Tach/V-Fib:	___	CHB:	_
		SV Arrhythmia:	___		

Other Complications: ___

Post Card Syndrome:	___	Pulmonary Embolus:	___
Hematoma:	___	Acute Renal Failure:	___
Pulmonary Insuff:	___	Acute Pulmonary Failure:	___
Diverticulitis:	___	Cholecystitis:	___
Pancreatitis:	___	Anticoagulant Comp:	___
GI Complications:	___	Pneumonia:	___
Unstable Sternum:	___	Tracheostomy:	___
Pericarditis:	___	Pneumothorax:	___
Diabetes Mellitus:	___	Tamponade:	___
Thrombophlebitis:	___	Pericardial Effusion:	___
Pericardial Tamponade:	___	DIC:	___
Vascular Comp:	___		

Other: ____

MORTALITY DATA

Mortality: ___

Date of Death: __-__-__ Days Survived: _____

Death Witnessed: ___ Autopsy: ___

Cause of Death: ____________________

Comments: ____________________________________

CARDIOPULMONARY TRANSPLANTATION REGISTRY
FOLLOWUP DATA

Patient Name (Press "Ctrl N"): .______________________________

Date of FollowUp: __-__-__ **BOSS #:** ____________

Hospital Admission: ___ **Date Of Admission:** __-__-__
Date Of Discharge: __-__-__ **LOS:** ___

Primary Diagnosis: ______________________

Physical Data: Height: ___ in ___ cm
Weight: ___ lb ____ kg
BP: ___ / ___
Heart Rate: ___

Condition: Hepatic ___ S3 ___ S4 ___
Rales ___ NVD ___ Edema ___
Cyanosis ___ Other ______________

Cardiac Rehab: ___ Rehab Center: ______________________

Predominant Symptoms:
Asymptomatic ___ Chest Pain ___
Dyspnea at Rest ___ Dyspnea on Exertion ___
Edema ___ Fatigue ___
Syncope ___ Palpitations ___
Near Syncope ___ SOB ___
Arrhythmia ___ Other ________________

NYHA Class: ___

Medications:

Medication Changes: ___

	Drugs	Dose	Frq	Date Start	Date Stop	Side Effects	Comments
1.				- -	- -	_	
2.				- -	- -	_	
3.				- -	- -	_	
4.				- -	- -	_	
5.				- -	- -	_	
6.				- -	- -	_	
7.				- -	- -	_	
8.				- -	- -	_	
9.				- -	- -	_	
10.				- -	- -	_	
11.				- -	- -	_	

POST-TRANSPLANT TESTS

Exercise: ___ **Date:** ___-___-___ **Protocol:** ______________

	Heart Rate	BP	Oxygen Uptake
Resting	___	___/___	_____ ml/min/k
Exercise	___	___/___	_____ ml/min/k

ST Segment Depression: ___ ____ mm

Leads: I ___ II ___ III ___

ECG: ___ Date: ___-___-___ Rhythm: ____________________

LVH	___	LBBB	___	RBBB	___
IVCD	___	SCAR	___	PM	___

SCAR:

Anterior	___	Inferior	___
Inferior-Post	___	Anterior-Lat	___
Lateral	___	Posterior	___

Other Abnormalities:

Subendocard Ischemia	___	ST-T Wave Abnormal	___
Poor R-Wave progress	___	Low Voltage L.Leads	___
Atrial Premature Beat	___	Vent Premature Beats	___

HB 1 ___ HB 2 ___ HB 3 ___

Holter: ___ Date: ___-___-___ Indication: ______________________

Previously Documented Arrhythmias: ___
Type: ____________
____
____

Permanent Pacemaker: ___ Type: ______________________

Abnormalities: ___ Symptoms: ___

Atrial:	______________	Ventricular:	______________
HB:	______________	PM Function:	______________
Sinus:	______________		

Comments: ____

Cardiac Ultrasound: ___ **Date:** __-__-__

M-Mode Echo: ___

		cm
RV Diameter	(Diastole)	____
LV Diameter	(Diastole)	____
LV Diameter	(Systole)	____
Septal Thickness	(Diastole)	____
LV Post Wall Thk	(Diastole)	____
Left Atrial Diameter	(Systole)	____
Aortic Root Diameter		____

2D/Doppler Echo: ___
Findings: ______________________________

SCANS

	Procedure	Date	Prim Dx	Sec Dx
1.	____________	__-__-__	____________	____________
	Comment:	____________		
2.	____________	__-__-__	____________	____________
	Comment:	____________		
3.	____________	__-__-__	____________	____________
	Comment:	____________		
4.	____________	__-__-__	____________	____________
	Comment:	____________		
5.	____________	__-__-__	____________	____________
	Comment:	____________		
6.	____________	__-__-__	____________	____________
	Comment:	____________		
7.	____________	__-__-__	____________	____________
	Comment:	____________		
8.	____________	__-__-__	____________	____________
	Comment:	____________		

Pulmonary Function: ___ Date: __-__-__

		Pre-Rx		% Pred
Spirometry:	FEV1	_____	L	___
	FEV1/FVC	_____	%	___
	FEF@%-75%	_____	L/sec	___
Lung Volumes:	VC	_____	L	___
	RV	_____	L	___
	RV/TLC	_____	%	___
Diffusion:	DLCO	_____	ml/min/mmHg	___

Cardiac Catheterization: ___ **Date:** __-__-__

Scheduling: __________

Indications: 1. ____________________
2. ____________________

Physical Dimensions: **Height (cm):** _____

Weight (kg): _____

BSA (M2): _____

Hemodynamic Data:	----Baseline-----		---Intervention---	
	Pressure (mm)	O2 Sat (%)	Pressure (mm)	O2 Sat (%)
Heart Rate (ppm)	___		___	
AO	___/___	____	___/___	____
LV	___/___	____	___/___	____
LA	V:___ M:___	____	V:___ M:___	____
PCW	V:___ M:___	____	V:___ M:___	____
PA	___/___	____	___/___	____
RV	___/___	____	___/___	____
RA	V:___ M:___	____	V:___ M:___	____
SVC	___/___	____	___/___	____
IVC	___/___	____	___/___	____

O2 Consumption (ml/min): _____
Hgb (gm): ____
Systemic AVO2 Difference (Vol %): _____
Pulmonary AVO2 Difference (Vol %): _____
Systemic Blood Flow (L/min): ____
Pulmonary Blood Flow (L/min): ____
Cardiac Index (L/min/M2): _____
Shunts: ____________________

Resistance (Wood Units):	Baseline	Intervention
SVR	____	____
PVR	____	____
TPR	____	____

Left Ventriculogram:

Segment	Contraction Pattern
Anterobasal	________________
Anterolateral	________________
Apical	________________
Diaphragmatic	________________
Posterobasal	________________
Basal Septal	________________
Apical Septal	________________
Posterolateral	________________
Inferior Lateral	________________
Superior Lateral	________________

Mitral Prolapse: ___ Mitral Regurg: _______

LV Volumes: EDV: _______ EDVI: _______
ESV: _______ ESVI: _______
SV: _______ SVI: _______

Ejection Fraction: ___

Regurgitation Fraction: ____

Aortogram: Aorta: ____________________
Aortic Valve: ____________
Aortic Regurg: ________

Remarks: ____

Coronary Angiography:

Coronary Artery	% Stenosis	Morphology Lesion	Morphology Segment	Collat Send	Notes
RCA prox	___	___________	___________	___	______
RCA mid	___	___________	___________	___	______
RCA dist	___	___________	___________	___	______
RPDA	___	___________	___________	___	______
RAV	___	___________	___________	___	______
RPL 1	___	___________	___________	___	______
RPL 2	___	___________	___________	___	______
RPL 3	___	___________	___________	___	______
Inf Sept	___	___________	___________	___	______
Ac Marg	___	___________	___________	___	______

LMCA	___	___	___	___	___
LAD prox	___	___	___	___	___
LAD mid	___	___	___	___	___
LAD dist	___	___	___	___	___
D1	___	___	___	___	___
D2	___	___	___	___	___
S1	___	___	___	___	___
Cx prox	___	___	___	___	___
Cx dist	___	___	___	___	___
OM1	___	___	___	___	___
OM2	___	___	___	___	___
OM3	___	___	___	___	___
LAV	___	___	___	___	___
LPL	___	___	___	___	___
LPDA	___	___	___	___	___
Other ______	___	___	___	___	___

Biopsy: ___

Date of Biposy: ___-___-___

Findings: ______________________

Indication:

Routine	___	Const Symptoms	___
Arrhythmia	___	Dyspnea	___
Cough	___	Edema	___
Hypotension	___	CHF	___
Fever	___	Other ___________	

Comments: ____

Treatment: ___

Hospitalized: ___

In/Outpatient:

IV Steroids: (1 Gm IV OD x 3) ---- ___

Increased Prednisone: (100 mg po x 5 days) ---- ___

High Dose Prednisone Taper: (1 mg/kg/day x 3 weeks)---- ___

OKT3: -- ___

Inpatient Only:

IV Steroids & ATGam: (3 or more days) ---- ___

ATGam: --- ___

Other Treatment: ______________________

Comments: ____

Blood Chemistries: ___

Liver Function:	**ALT**	_____	**AST**	_____
	Alk Ph	_____	**Total Bili**	_____
	Total Protein	_____	**Albumin**	_____
Lipids:	**Cholesterol**	_____	**Triglycerides**	_____
	HDL	_____	**LDL**	_____
Hematology:	**WBC**	_____	**Hgb**	_____
	Hct	_____	**Platelets**	_______
Electrolytes:	**Sodium (Na)**	_____	**Potassium (K)**	_____
	Chloride (Cl)	_____	**CO2**	_____
Glucose:	_____	**Fasting:** ___		

Renal Function: ___

BUN (mg/dl): _____ Creatinine (mg/dl): _____
Creat Clearance: _____
Total Volume: _____

Cyclosporine Levels:

RIA: ______
HPLC: ______

Comments: ____

Complications: ___

Type: __________________________

Infection: ___	Date	Source	Organism	Treatment
Bacterial ___	- -	______	______	______
Fungus ___	- -	______	______	______
Viral ___	- -	______	______	______
Other ______	- -	______	______	______

Viral Titers: CMV: 1:______ EBV: 1:______ TOXO: 1:______

Viral Antibodies: CMV: ___ EBV: ___ HAA: ___ HIV: ___ TOXO: _

Comments: ____
____
____

POST TRANSPLANT SURGICAL PROCEDURES

Organ	Procedure	Diagnosis	Date
___	___	___	__-__-__
Outcome: ___			
___	___	___	__-__-__
Outcome: ___			
___	___	___	__-__-__
Outcome: ___			
___	___	___	__-__-__
Outcome: ___			
___	___	___	__-__-__
Outcome: ___			

Comments: ___

Immunization: ___

Next Scheduled Biopsy: __-__-__

Next Scheduled Annual Visit: __-__-__

Index